ECG Interpretation in Equine Practice

ECG Interpretation in Equine Practice

Katharyn Jean Mitchell
BVSc, DVCS, DVM, PhD, Diplomate ACVIM (LAIM)
Clinic for Equine Internal Medicine
Swiss Equine Cardiology Consulting
Equine Department
University of Zurich
Zurich
Switzerland

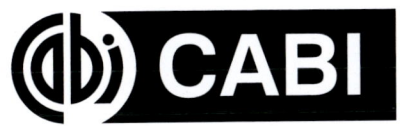

CABI is a trading name of CAB International

CABI
Nosworthy Way
Wallingford
Oxfordshire OX10 8DE
UK

Tel: +44 (0)1491 832111
Fax: +44 (0)1491 833508
E-mail: info@cabi.org
Website: www.cabi.org

CABI
745 Atlantic Avenue
8th Floor
Boston, MA 02111
USA

Tel: +1 (617)682-9015
E-mail: cabi-nao@cabi.org

A catalogue record for this book is available from the British Library, London, UK.

References to Internet websites (URLs) were accurate at the time of writing.

ISBN-13: 9781789240825 (paperback)
9781789240832 (ePDF)
9781789240849 (ePub)

Commissioning Editor: Alexandra Lainsbury
Editorial Assistant: Emma McCann
Production Editor: James Bishop

Front cover photograph courtesy Meredith Flash-O'neil
Typeset by SPi, Pondicherry, India
Printed and bound by CPI Group (UK) Ltd, Croydon, CR0 4YY

Foreword

From early on in my life, I was interested in cardiology. One of the first books I purchased as a veterinary student was on ECG reading in small animals because no such book was available for practitioners with an equine focus. The aim of this book, *ECG Interpretation in Equine Practice*, is to fill that gap and provide a hands-on guide for veterinarians to use when recording, diagnosing and treating arrhythmias in equine patients.

Advances in veterinary medical technology provide easier and more affordable access to ECG recording and transmitting equipment, making ECG recordings feasible in the field and in hospital settings. The recording of resting or exercising ECGs is now a common part of the diagnostic evaluation in horses with arrhythmias, poor performance or cardiac disease. In addition, newer pharmacological therapies and interventional techniques are available to treat equine patients with arrhythmias, and this field of equine cardiology research has rapidly expanded in the last 10 years. Further work is still required to understand fully the effects of arrhythmias on performance and to describe accurately the risk of adverse events in equine patients with arrhythmias. We will continue working in this area to help advance the field of equine cardiology.

I hope that this book will be helpful and frequently utilized by equine practitioners when examining equine patients with arrhythmias.

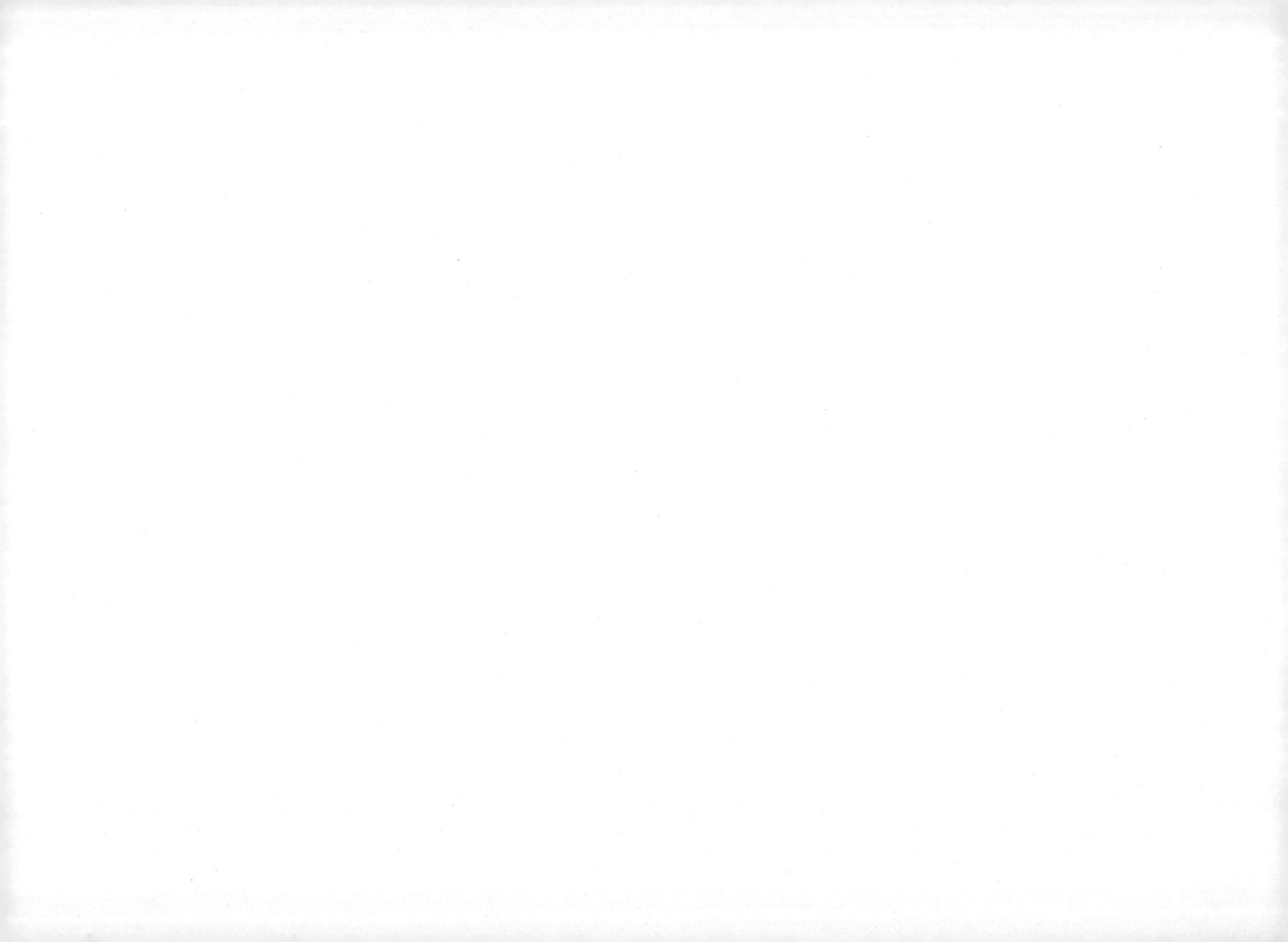

Acknowledgements

To my family: thank you for all your love and support, particularly to my mum Cherrie Mitchell for instilling a love of cardiology in me from an early age.

To Professor Colin Schwarzwald: thank you for the opportunity to learn equine cardiology.

To my patients and their owners: thank you for the opportunity to explore equine cardiology and learn about electrophysiology in the most practical way possible. Without you, none of this would be possible.

Contents

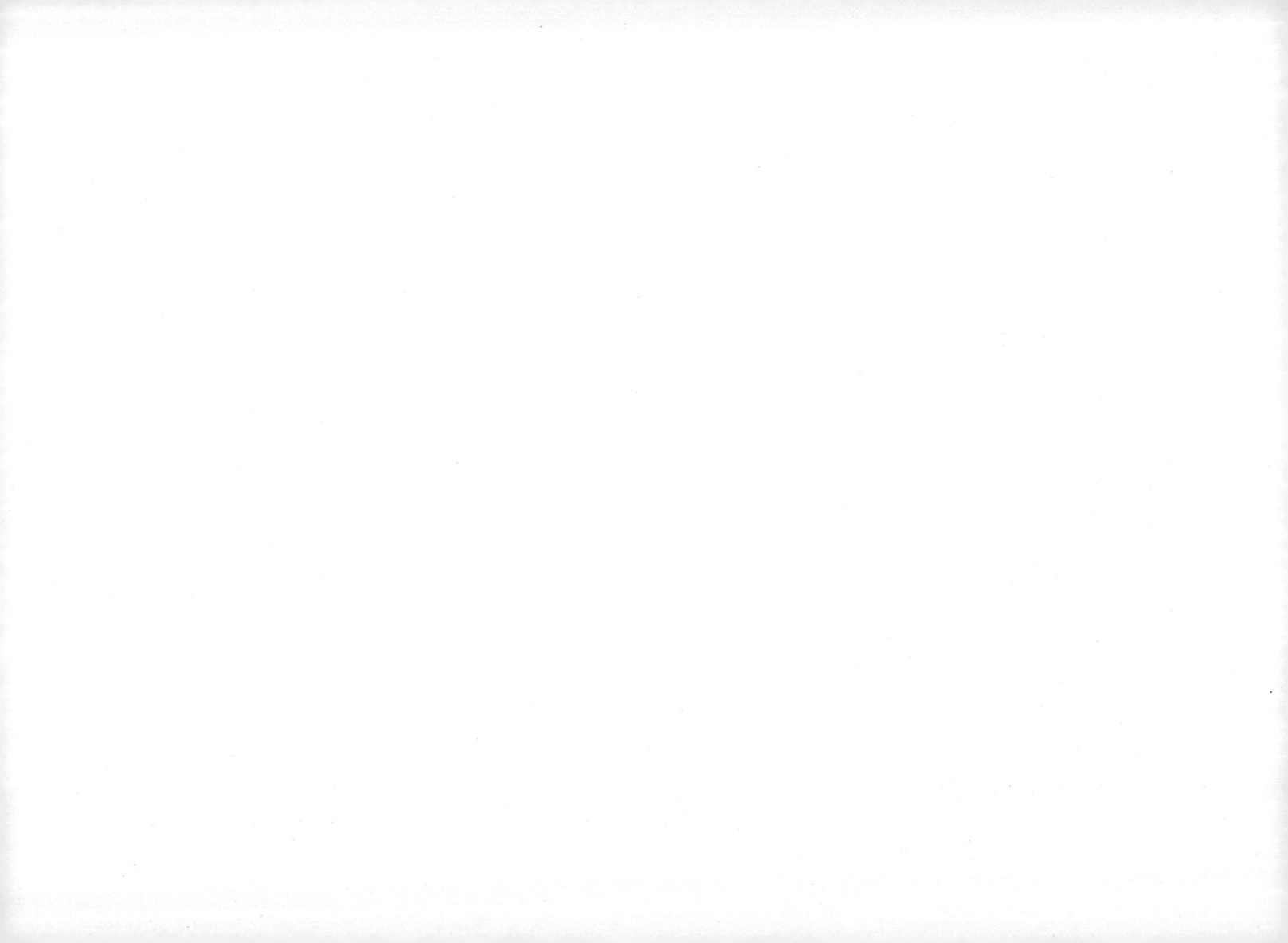

Basics of Electrocardiography

What is an ECG?

A surface electrocardiogram (ECG) is a graphical representation of the sum of electrical signals produced by the cardiomyocytes during the cardiac cycle. Electrodes attached to the skin are used to detect these signals, which are then transferred by cables to an electrocardiograph, where the signals are filtered, amplified and printed directly on paper or displayed on a screen. Recording an ECG is essential for diagnosing both arrhythmias and conduction disturbances.

Indications for Obtaining an ECG Recording in Horses

In horses, ECGs are required to obtain a definitive diagnosis when an abnormal heart rate or rhythm has been detected on physical examination (Box 1.1).

Electrical Properties of the Equine Myocardium

The generation of an action potential in both nodal and ventricular myocardial tissue is explained in Fig. 1.1. The cell-to-cell propagation of these action potentials results in depolarization (and subsequent repolarization) of larger areas of myocardial tissue, which in turn are detected during a surface ECG recording (Opie, 1998; Bers, 2002).

- When an arrhythmia is heard on physical examination.
- When horses have unexplained tachyarrhythmias or bradyarrhythmias.
- In the evaluation of horses with exercise intolerance or poor performance.
- In the evaluation of horses with evidence of moderate to severe structural heart disease potentially predisposing to the development of arrhythmias.
- In the evaluation of horses with a history of weakness or collapse.
- To confirm normal sinus rhythm is present during a pre-purchase examination.
- When monitoring heart rhythm as part of therapy (e.g. anti-arrhythmic therapy).
- When monitoring heart rate to detect stress or pain (e.g. during a hospital stay or transport).
- When monitoring a horse during sedation or general anaesthesia.
- When monitoring a horse that is critically ill (e.g. electrolyte imbalance, intoxication).

Fig. 1.1. (A) Phases of the action potential (AP) occurring in a typical ventricular cardiomyocyte. There are four phases of the AP, with rapid entry of sodium (Na^+) ions into the cell resulting in fast depolarization (phase 0) and calcium (Ca^{2+}) ions entering more slowly during phase 2, resulting in full depolarization of the cell. Potassium (K^+) channels open, and outward movement of K^+ ions accounts for repolarization of the cell (phases 1 and 3). Phase 4, the maintenance of the resting membrane potential in a state of polarization, results from K^+ diffusing out of the cell following the concentration gradient that is maintained by the Na^+/K^+-ATPase (see panel C). (B) Timing of the movement of ions across the cellular membrane, resulting in the phases of the AP seen in panel (A). (C) Phases of the AP occurring in a typical pacemaker cell (e.g. sino-atrial or atrioventricular node). Here, these cells have a lower resting membrane potential than other cardiomyocytes, with the cell becoming steadily more positive during phase 4 due to slow Ca^{2+} influx through Ca^{2+} channels, eventually resulting in spontaneous Ca^{2+}-driven depolarization. Note that the slope of phase 0 is flatter (i.e. slower) than that of the ventricular AP. This spontaneous depolarization of nodal tissue is known as automaticity. (D) A stylized cardiomyocyte, depicting examples of ion pumps, channels and exchangers that allow the movement of ions across the cell membrane, resulting in depolarization and repolarization of the cell membrane. The Na^+/K^+-ATPase is primarily responsible for maintaining the resting intracellular concentrations of ions (high intracellular K^+, low intracellular Na^+). Opening of the Na^+ channels results in rapid influx of Na^+ during early depolarization. Calcium ions enter the cell during the AP through Ca^{2+} channels, leading to a Ca^{2+}-induced Ca^{2+} release from the sarcoendoplasmic reticulum (SER) and subsequent contraction of actin and myosin filaments. The excess cytoplasmic Ca^{2+} is then either eliminated by re-uptake into the SER or removed from the cell via the Na^+/Ca^{2+} exchanger and a Ca^{2+}-ATPase pump. There are several different K^+ channels that allow K^+ to exit the cell during repolarization and the resting state. (Adapted from Mitchell, 2019, with permission.)

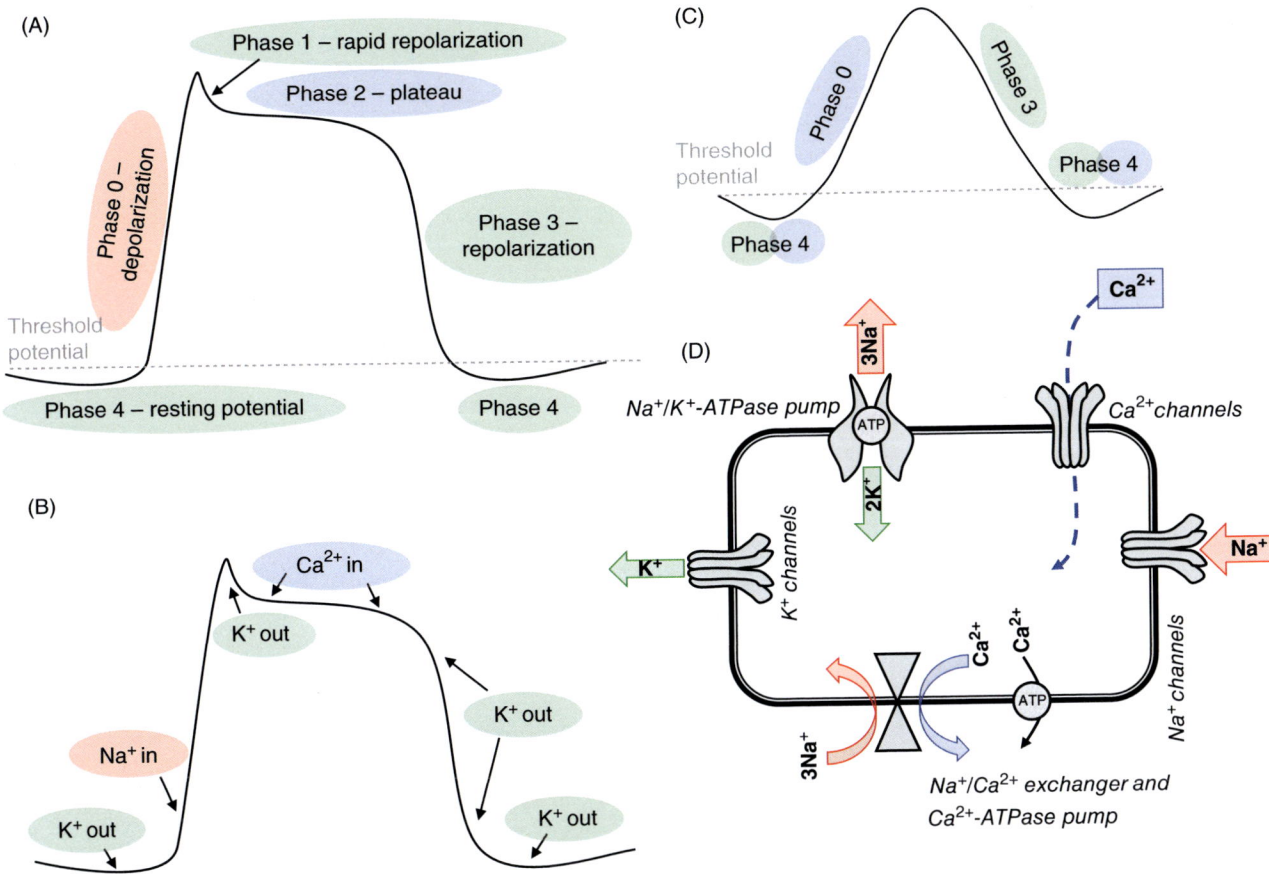

Fig. 1.1.

Normal Cardiac Conduction and Components of P-QRS-T Complexes

In horses, the conduction of electrical activity across the heart follows a fairly fixed pathway from the sinoatrial (SA) node, across the atrial myocardium, through the atrioventricular (AV) node and then down the bundle of His, bundle branches and Purkinje system to the ventricular myocardium. The spontaneously depolarizing regular rhythm generated from the SA node is known as 'normal sinus rhythm'. This normal conduction pattern and resulting surface ECG is illustrated in Fig. 1.2.

For the depolarization or repolarization to be accurately detected on a surface ECG, a relatively large amount of myocardial tissue is required for activation. Therefore, the sinus depolarizations are not visualized per se; rather, it is the spread of depolarization across the atria creating the P wave that is seen on the ECG. The morphology of the P waves is highly variable between and within horses, with bifid (two positive peaks), single-positive or biphasic (typically negative/positive) waves commonly observed, even within the same ECG trace (Fig. 1.3A). As heart rate fluctuates, the P-wave morphology may change, while some horses display evidence of a wandering pacemaker within the large SA node, particularly at low heart rates (i.e. with high parasympathetic tone), resulting in highly variable P-wave morphology between individual beats. After atrial depolarization, there is a period of atrial repolarization, which can occasionally be seen on a surface ECG as a so-called T_a wave (i.e. the atrial T wave), as seen in Fig. 1.3B.

Fig. 1.2. (A) The impulse generation and conduction system within the myocardium and (B) a base–apex surface ECG recording resulting from impulse conduction through the different segments of the conduction system. The impulse initiates in the sinoatrial node (SAN) and is transmitted across the atrial myocardium, generating the P wave (B; blue line). Specialized internodal and interatrial (Bachmann's bundle) pathways facilitate and direct impulse conduction within the atria. At the atrioventricular node (AVN), impulse conduction is delayed, resulting in the PR interval (B; yellow line) observed on the surface ECG. Rapid conduction then occurs through the bundle of His, bundle branches and Purkinje fibre network, activating the ventricular myocardium and generating the QRS complex (B; red line) on the ECG. CrVCa, cranial vena cava; RA, right atrium; LA, left atrium; H, bundle of His; RV, right ventricle; LV, left ventricle. (From Mitchell, 2019, with permission. Adapted from van Loon, G. and Patteson, M. (2010) Electrophysiology and arrhythmogenesis. In: Marr, C.M. (ed.) *Cardiology of the Horse*. 2nd edn. Elsevier, pp. 59–73; and from Schwarzwald, C.C., Bonagura, J.D. and Muir, W.W. (2009) The cardiovascular system. In: Muir, W.W. (ed.) *Equine Anaesthesia*, 2nd edn. Elsevier, pp. 37–100, with permission.)

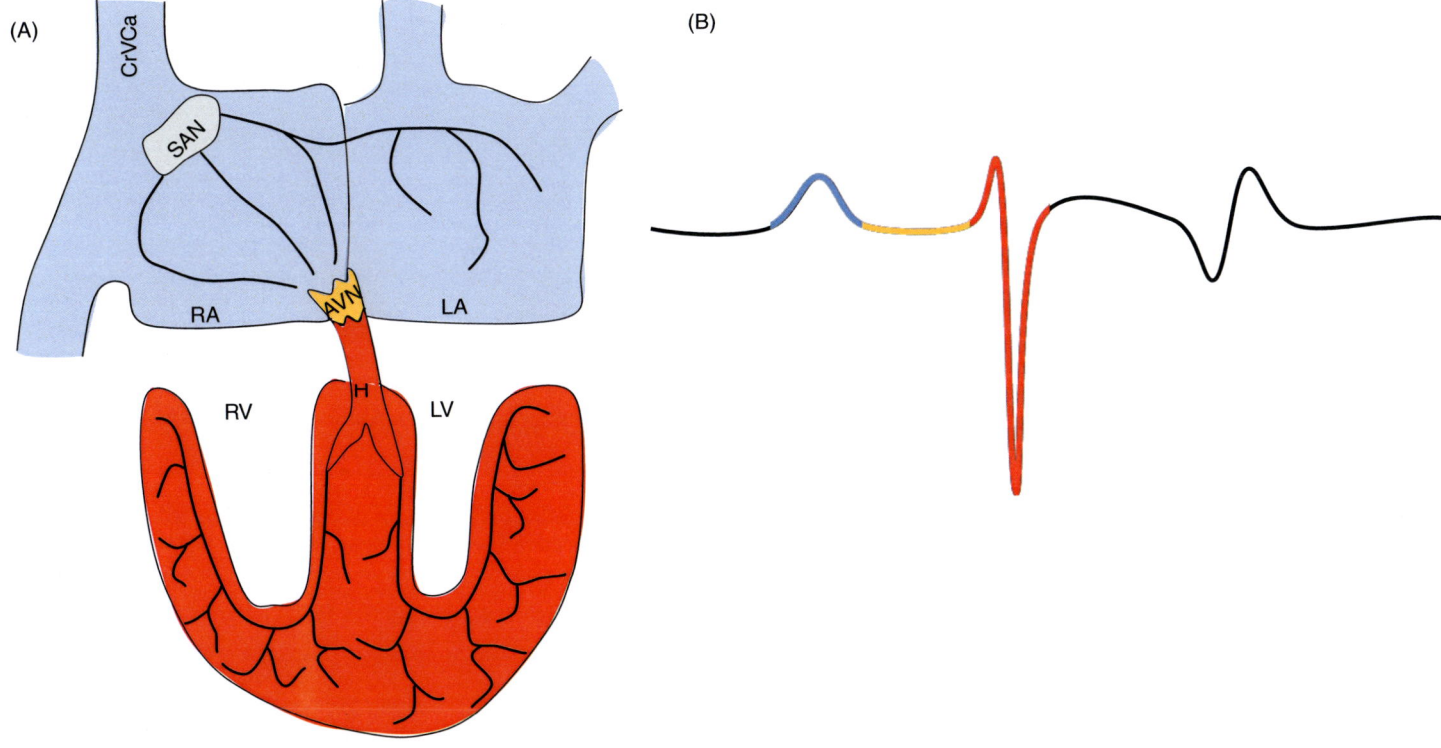

Fig. 1.2.

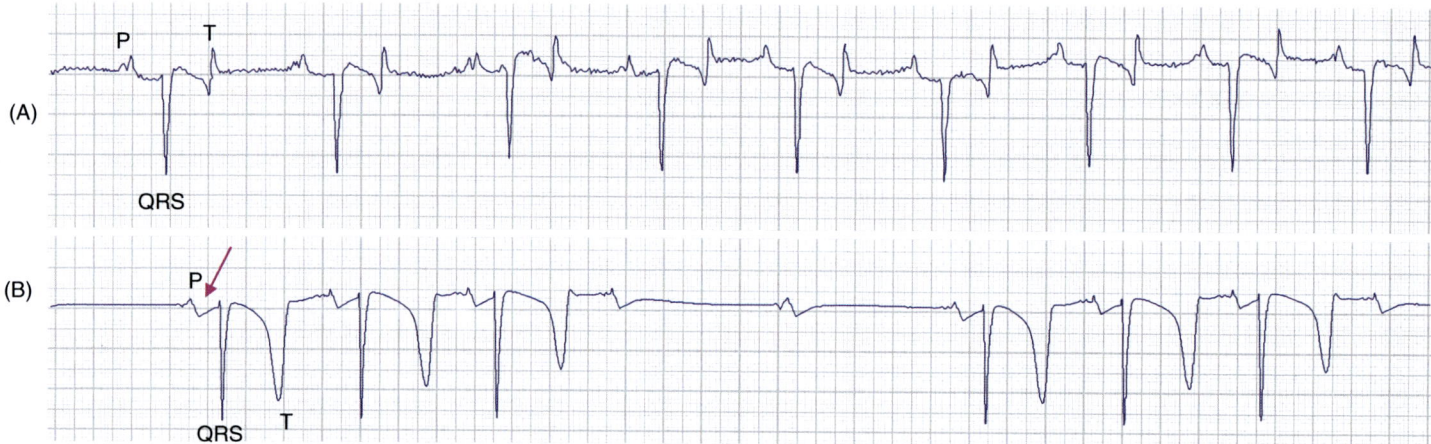

Fig. 1.3. (A) Typical P-QRS-T complex morphology from a healthy horse, as recorded with a standard base–apex lead configuration, selecting lead I to be displayed. Variable (from bifid to monophasic) P-wave morphology is observed with increasing heart rate. The ventricular depolarization has an S morphology, while the T waves are biphasic (negative–positive). Paper speed: 25 mm/s. (B) A base–apex ECG lead II recording from a horse with second-degree atrioventricular blocks. The atrial repolarization (T_a wave, purple arrow) is observed as a negative depression following the P wave. The P waves have similar morphology; the ventricular depolarization has an S morphology, while the T waves are negative. Paper speed: 25 mm/s.

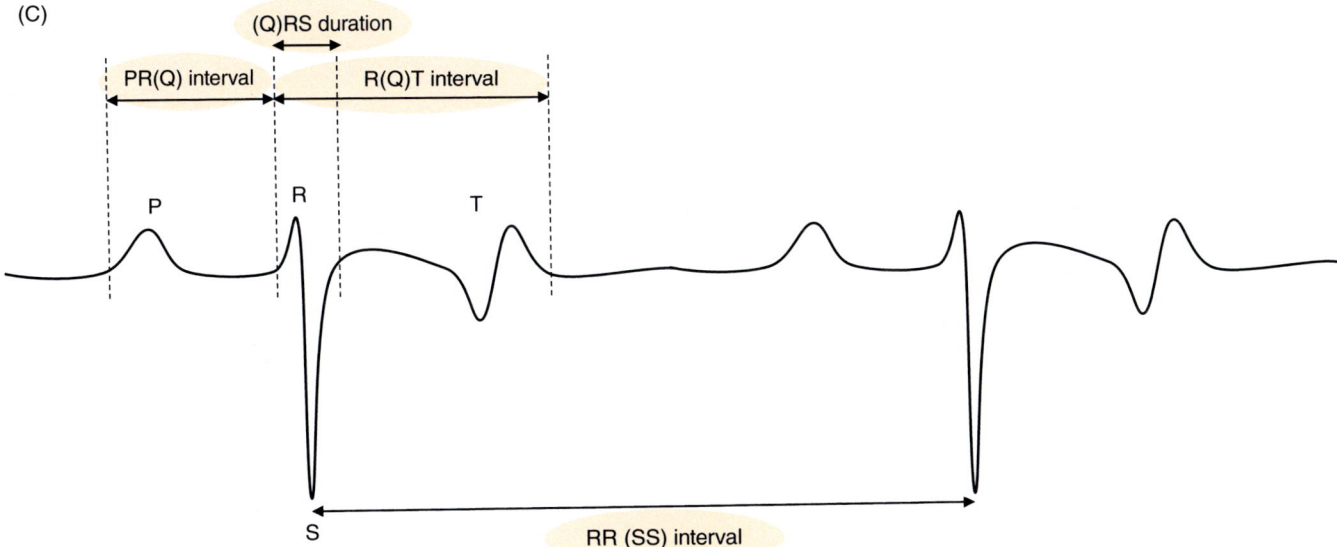

(C)

Fig. 1.3. Continued.

(C) The important ECG timing intervals are indicated. The equine base–apex lead ECG does not typically have identifiable Q waves. Therefore, the conventional nomenclature of the timing intervals may require modification – the PQ interval becomes the PR interval, the QRS duration is the RS duration and the QT interval is actually the RT interval. Because the largest deflection of the equine QRS is negative – this is called the S wave – so the interval measured between adjacent QRS intervals is actually the SS interval, rather than the RR interval. However, in most instances, for simplicity and consistency across species, the intervals are still called PQ, QRS, QT and RR intervals. Note that it can be difficult to accurately define the start and end of the individual deflections. When measuring timing intervals, it can be helpful to increase the paper speed (e.g. from 25 to 50 or 100 mm/s), maintain a standardized approach (e.g. always measure from the onset or end of the deflection where it deviates clearly from the baseline) and limit the number of observers (i.e. ideally, the same person should perform the analysis if repeated measurements over time are required). (Adapted from Mitchell, 2019, with permission.)

In a normal equine heart, the atria and ventricles are electrically separated from each other by non-conducting fibrous tissue, except at the level of the AV node. Conduction of the electrical impulse through the AV node is slower than through the other myocardial tissues, resulting in a delay between the atrial and ventricular depolarization. This is physiologically important because it allows the atrial contribution to ventricular filling to occur before the onset of ventricular systole, optimizing pre-load and therefore cardiac output. Healthy horses commonly have high parasympathetic (vagal) tone, which can further slow (or even block) AV nodal conduction. Conduction through the AV node does not result in a deflection on the surface ECG, but the conduction delay can be measured through the PR interval (as seen in Figs 1.2B and 1.3C).

Once the impulse has travelled through the AV node, it moves rapidly through the bundle of His, bundle branches and Purkinje fibre system to depolarize the ventricular myocardium. This near-simultaneous depolarization of a large amount of myocardial tissue results in the largest deflections recorded on the surface ECG – the QRS complex. According to international convention, the first downward deflection is the Q wave, the first upward deflection is the R wave and the next following downward deflection is the S wave. The larger waves are denoted in capitals, while the smaller waves are denoted in lower-case letters. Typically, horses have an rS or S morphology when an ECG is recorded using a base–apex lead configuration (Fig. 1.3). Q waves are rarely identified on equine surface base–apex ECG recordings. Despite the largest wave of the typical equine QRS complex being the S wave, rather than the R wave as in standard human or small-animal ECGs, for convention, we still refer to the interval between two adjacent QRS complexes as the RR interval.

Every depolarization *must* be followed by repolarization; therefore *every* QRS complex is *always* followed by a T wave (representing repolarization). Horses have extremely labile T-wave morphology, with variations in polarity and duration highly dependent on parasympathetic tone and heart rate. Changes in T-wave morphology should not be overinterpreted in the diagnosis of cardiac disease; however, they can be helpful when determining the presence of abnormal complexes (atrial or ventricular premature complexes) and distinguishing artefacts (which do not have T waves) (Broux *et al.*, 2016).

Recognition of the normal equine P-QRS-T morphology is critical in assessing an equine ECG recording, and particular attention should be paid to the polarity of waveforms (particularly QRS-T) and the timing intervals. As equine ECGs are commonly missing the Q wave, the conventional timing intervals applied from human medicine require modification. The PQ interval becomes the PR interval, the QRS duration becomes the RS duration and the QT interval becomes the RT interval, although the conventional nomenclature is often referred to for simplicity. These timing intervals are illustrated in Fig. 1.3C and described in Table 1.1. When measuring the time intervals (PR(Q) interval, (Q)RS duration and R(Q)T interval), the size of the horse should be considered, as body weight is directly correlated with the time intervals (i.e. small horses generally have shorter time intervals) (Schwarzwald *et al.*, 2012).

Table 1.1. ECG timing intervals (mean and 95% confidence intervals) for a 500 kg horse at rest. (Data derived from Schwarzwald *et al.*, 2012.)

	Mean	95% Confidence Interval
Heart rate (bpm)	40	25–55
RR interval (ms)	1500	1050–2100
PR interval (ms)	300	200–380
QRS duration (ms)	115	85–145
QT$_{uncorrected}$ interval (ms)	480	400–580

It is important to note that, due to the extensive Purkinje fibre system within the equine ventricular myocardium (compared with humans and small animals), the equine QRS complex recorded from a typical base–apex lead configuration provides no reliable information about cardiac chamber size. Therefore, equine ECGs should not be used for the diagnosis of cardiac hypertrophy or dilation; however, echocardiography can provide useful information about myocardial changes (Hamlin and Smith, 1965).

ECG Lead Terminology

Electrodes placed on the body surface are used to measure changes in the electrical potential created during myocardial depolarization and repolarization. A combination of two electrodes (one negative and one positive) creates a 'lead'. When electrodes are placed across the surface of the body around the heart, the sum of all electrical potentials can be recorded. Movement of the electrical signal towards a positive electrode will create an upward deflection on the ECG, while movement away from a positive electrode will result in a downward deflection on the ECG tracing.

In the horse, many of the standard human or small-animal ECG lead placements are not commonly utilized due to the impracticality of placing multiple limb and chest leads on a large moving object. However, many of the electrodes and ECG recorders are still labelled for conventional human or small-animal use (i.e. right arm (RA), left arm (LA), left leg or foot (LL)).

Typically, most equine ECGs are recorded utilizing the principles of Einthoven's triangle, the most simple being a 'base–apex' or three-lead configuration as described in Table 1.2. The RA electrode is placed on the right caudal neck while the LA and LL electrodes are placed on the left thorax at the heart apex (Fig. 1.4). Lead I (recorded between the RA and LA electrodes) and lead II (recorded between the RA and LL electrodes) will produce similar ECG morphology when used in this configuration (Fig. 1.3A).

Twelve-lead ECGs (as opposed to a single-lead base–apex ECG or a traditional limb-lead ECG) provide a larger variety of projections of the heart's electrical activity and have the potential to help determine the origin of premature complexes in horses. However, respective criteria for assessment have not been established so far and work is currently ongoing in this area (van Steenkiste *et al.*, 2018).

Table 1.2. Standard base–apex electrode positioning in the horse.

ECG electrode	Position
Neutral/earth	If present, can be placed anywhere
Right arm (RA)	Right caudal neck
Left arm (LA)	Left heart apex
Left leg/foot (LL)	Left heart apex

Fig. 1.4. Positioning of the ECG electrodes to obtain a standard base–apex lead from a resting horse, useful for obtaining short-term ECG recordings. The electrode positions described by Einthoven's triangle are modified and positioned on the body of the horse. The right arm (RA) electrode is placed on the right neck of the horse, while the left arm (LA) and left leg (LL) electrodes are placed on the left side of the horse over the apex of the heart. With this electrode configuration, both 'lead I' (RA→LA) and 'lead II' (RA→LL) can be chosen on the ECG recorder to display the base–apex ECG trace. Note that the terminology (LA, RA and LL; lead I, II and III) originates from the Einthoven lead system.

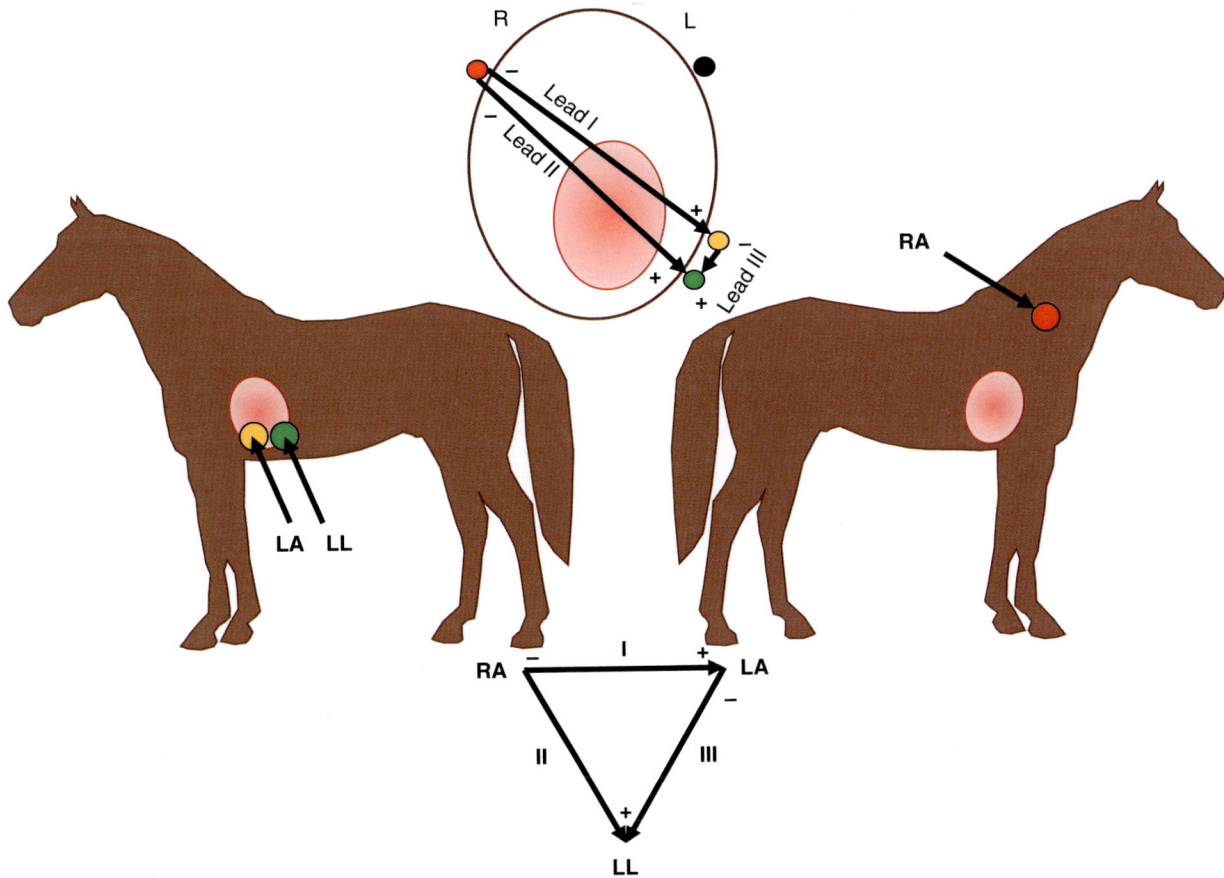

Fig. 1.4.

Recording an ECG

Equipment

The basic equipment required to obtain an ECG recording includes electrodes, a recording device and a display of the tracing (Box 2.1). A wide variety of point-of-care medical devices have been brought to the market in recent times, making ECG recording devices easier to use and more affordable for the equine practitioner.

Recording devices

ECG recordings of short duration can easily be obtained using hand-held devices (e.g. Alivecor Kardia Mobile ECG; Alivecor, Mountain View, California, USA) or a variety of common multi-purpose monitoring devices (e.g. Medtronic LIFEPAK 15 monitor/defibrillator; Physio-Control, Redmond, Washington, DC, USA). Equine-oriented, purpose-built ECG recorders (e.g. Televet 100 telemetric ECG system; Engel Engineering Services GmbH, Heusenstamm, Germany) are also readily available. Many of these devices display the ECG tracing on a monitor, smart phone or tablet computer. Each device must contain some type of storage capability, as an ECG recording is considered part of the medical record. This can be as simple as a thermoprinter providing hard copies of ECG strips of any length. Preferably, the device should save the data digitally, allowing the ECG to be post-processed, digitally analysed, interpreted, stored or sent to an expert for further analysis.

Extended, continuous recordings (e.g. longer than 5 min) require the use of a mobile device, which preferably records both locally (e.g. on an SD card) and remotely by sending the signal wirelessly (e.g. via Bluetooth or a mobile GSM network) to a storage device with

> **Box 2.1.** Basic equipment required to record an ECG
>
> - Electrodes (crocodile-style clip-on or self-adhesive gel-patch electrodes).
> - Electrical cables and recording device.
> - Display and recording system (direct print versus digital storage).

a display monitor (e.g. laptop, computer or smartphone, or a cloud-based server). For use in horses, the most commonly used veterinary device for this purpose is the Televet recorder, although many human or small-animal devices can be adapted for equine use (e.g. Lifecard CF; SpaceLab Healthcare, Snoqualmie, Washington, DC, USA). It is essential that the data from long-term ambulatory recordings are digitalized, stored and available for further offline processing and analysis. This also allows the easy sharing of ECG recordings between individuals, which can be useful when a second opinion is required.

Several products are currently in development to improve the quality and ease of ECG recording in horses, particularly during exercise. However, at this time, the Televet recorder is most commonly utilized and, in the author's opinion, remains the most reliable and easy-to-use product. It should be noted that the (veterinary) medical technology market has a number of heart-rate monitors currently available, but these should not be confused with an ECG recording device. Heart-rate monitors are supposed to detect RR intervals, but an unknown amount of post-processing occurs with the use of proprietary signal processing algorithms and filters to remove motion artefacts and arrhythmias. The accuracy and reliability of these devices cannot easily be verified by the user, and some of those tested have not provided accurate results in horses with arrhythmias or with exceptionally high heart rates during exercise (Lenoir *et al.*, 2017).

Heart-rate monitors provide no information on P-QRS-T morphology and are not considered a substitute for an ECG recorder in the diagnosis and management of equine arrhythmias. They can, however, be useful (acknowledging their limitations), particularly for monitoring heart rates during exercise at home with the owner.

Recently, the use of subcutaneous, implantable loop recorders (e.g. Reveal; Medtronic, Minneapolis, Minnesota, USA) in horses has shown encouraging preliminary results when used as event recorders over extended periods of time (weeks or months). These devices may be useful in patients with paroxysmal arrhythmias that occur infrequently, particularly when investigating horses with collapse. However, these devices are currently cost-prohibitive for most patients and require specific positioning to obtain an optimal ECG signal (Buhl, 2017; J. Keen, University of Edinburgh, 2017, personal communication).

Electrodes

Crocodile-style clip-on electrodes attached to ECG cables can be used to obtain short-term recordings. However, these are not suitable for longer-duration recordings, and some horses will not tolerate these, even for a short period of time. The application of water, normal saline or alcohol to the skin/crocodile clips is often required to ensure adequate contact and a good-quality ECG recording.

Self-adhesive gel-patch electrodes provide a more comfortable alternative to crocodile clips and can remain in place for several hours of recording without issue. For extended-duration (overnight) or exercising recordings, these sticky ECG electrodes can be further secured using self-adhesive foam patches (Fig. 2.1A) or an elastic bandage applied on top (Fig. 2.1D). In most cases, clipping the coat is unnecessary, as long as the gel patch remains moist and the self-adhesive part of the electrode stays dry and provides sufficient adhesive strength. Occasionally, with a thick winter (or Icelandic or donkey) coat, clipping small patches is necessary to provide better contact of the gel electrode with the skin surface. It is essential for the coat to be dry (e.g. before exercise) when the self-adhesive electrodes are applied, as they will not stick to a damp or wet surface.

Additional material

To obtain ambulatory recordings, it is necessary to affix the mobile recording/transmitting device to the horse. This is achieved using a reusable surcingle, purpose built for holding the device and the associated cables safely out of the way of damage, particularly if the horse lies down (e.g. Kruuse Televet Electrode Support; Jørgen Kruuse A/S, Langeskov, Denmark) (Fig. 2.1B, C). Alternatively, the device can be affixed using single-use sticky elastic bandages (Fig. 2.1D). Placement of appropriate padding over the withers region is important, particularly if the device is to be worn overnight or for several days.

Lead Placement

As discussed in Chapter 1, Fig. 1.4 shows the typical lead placement for a short-duration, resting ECG recording. This is considered a 'base–apex' configuration, where either lead I (RA→LA) or lead II (RA→LL) can be chosen on the monitor to display the ECG trace. Fig. 1.3A represents the typical P-QRS-T orientation when using this lead placement. Figure 2.2 displays the 'modified base–apex'

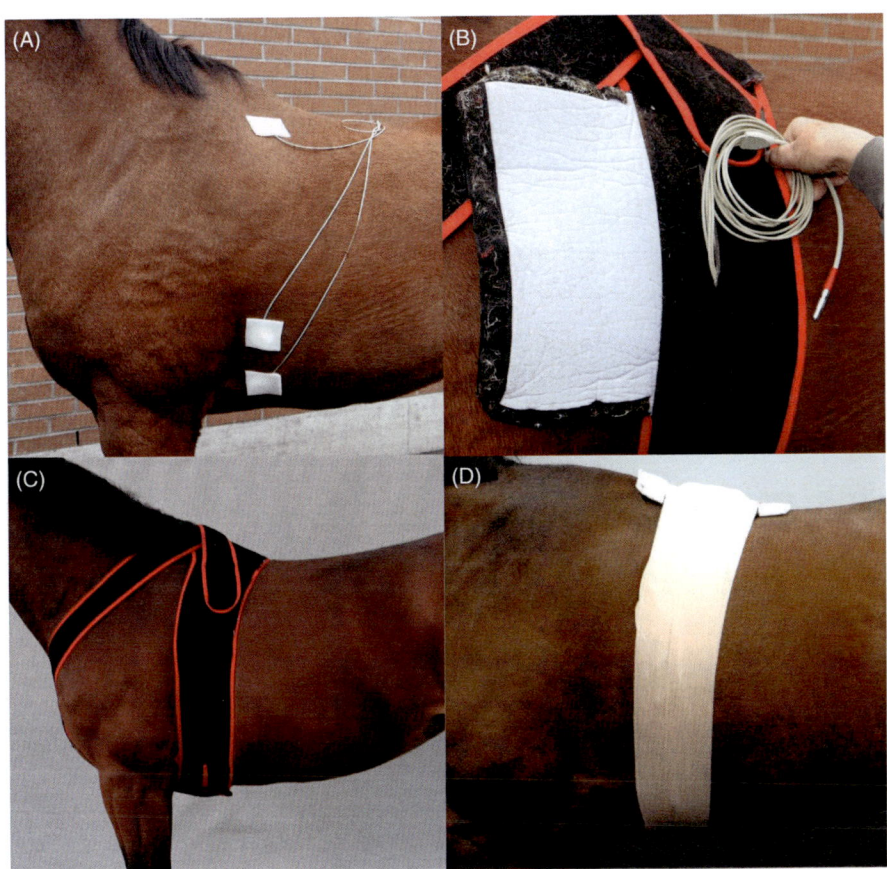

Fig. 2.1. (A) Self-adhesive gel-patch ECG electrodes and ECG cables covered with self-adhesive foam patches to further secure the electrodes and reduce artefacts. (B, C) A commercially available, reusable surcingle (Kruuse Televet Electrode Support; Jørgen Kruuse A/S, Langeskov, Denmark) can be used to secure the ECG electrodes, cables and transmitting device; this is useful for longer-duration or exercising ECG recordings. Pockets with Velcro are used to protect the cables and transmitting device while allowing easy access (e.g. for battery changes). (D) As an alternative, the ECG electrodes, cables and transmitting device can be secured with single-use, sticky elastic bandages. It is important that adequate padding is applied over the withers to avoid rubbing and pressure sores.

configuration that the author typically uses for longer-duration ambulatory ECG recordings. With this configuration, lead I will highlight the atrial electrical activity, producing slightly magnified P waves to aid in the differentiation of atrial ectopic complexes. Lead II will produce the typical ECG seen in Fig. 2.3. Lead III (LA→LL) will produce an alternative QRS configuration, which can aid in the detection of ventricular ectopic complexes.

During exercise, the ECG electrodes can remain in the same position as described above (Fig. 2.4A, B), resulting in the ECG seen in Fig. 2.5A, or can be moved to accommodate any equipment necessary (e.g. saddle, surcingle or harness). Figure 2.4C is a variation that the author uses particularly for lunging, treadmill or ridden exercise. The downside of this lead configuration is that lead I and lead II are very similar (Fig. 2.5B), which can make subtle changes in QRS configuration harder to identify but provides a 'back-up' lead in case one electrode becomes dislodged during exercise.

Resting ECG Recording

The criteria for determining the duration of a resting ECG recording are provided in Table 2.1.

Short-duration recordings

Shorter recordings can be easily obtained from well-restrained horses standing quietly. Many of the hand-held devices require the application of water, normal saline or alcohol to the skin to facilitate conduction of the signal. Movement artefacts frequently interfere with the recording quality and subsequent interpretation of the ECG findings, so care should be taken to ensure a good-quality recording is obtained.

Fig. 2.2. Positioning of the ECG electrodes to obtain a modified base–apex recording from a resting horse. This electrode configuration allows the three leads (right arm (RA) electrode, left arm (LA) electrode and left leg or foot (LL) electrode) to each highlight different aspects of cardiac depolarization/repolarization. This configuration is particularly useful for telemetric ECG monitoring or long-term (ambulatory, Holter) ECG recordings. In this example, the electrodes are coloured for use with the Televet 100 recording system. Note that the colour system corresponds to the International Electrotechnical Commison (IEC) standard; other devices may use a different colour system (i.e. the one defined by the American Heart Association, where RA is white, LA is black, N is green and LL is red). N, neutral/ground electrode.

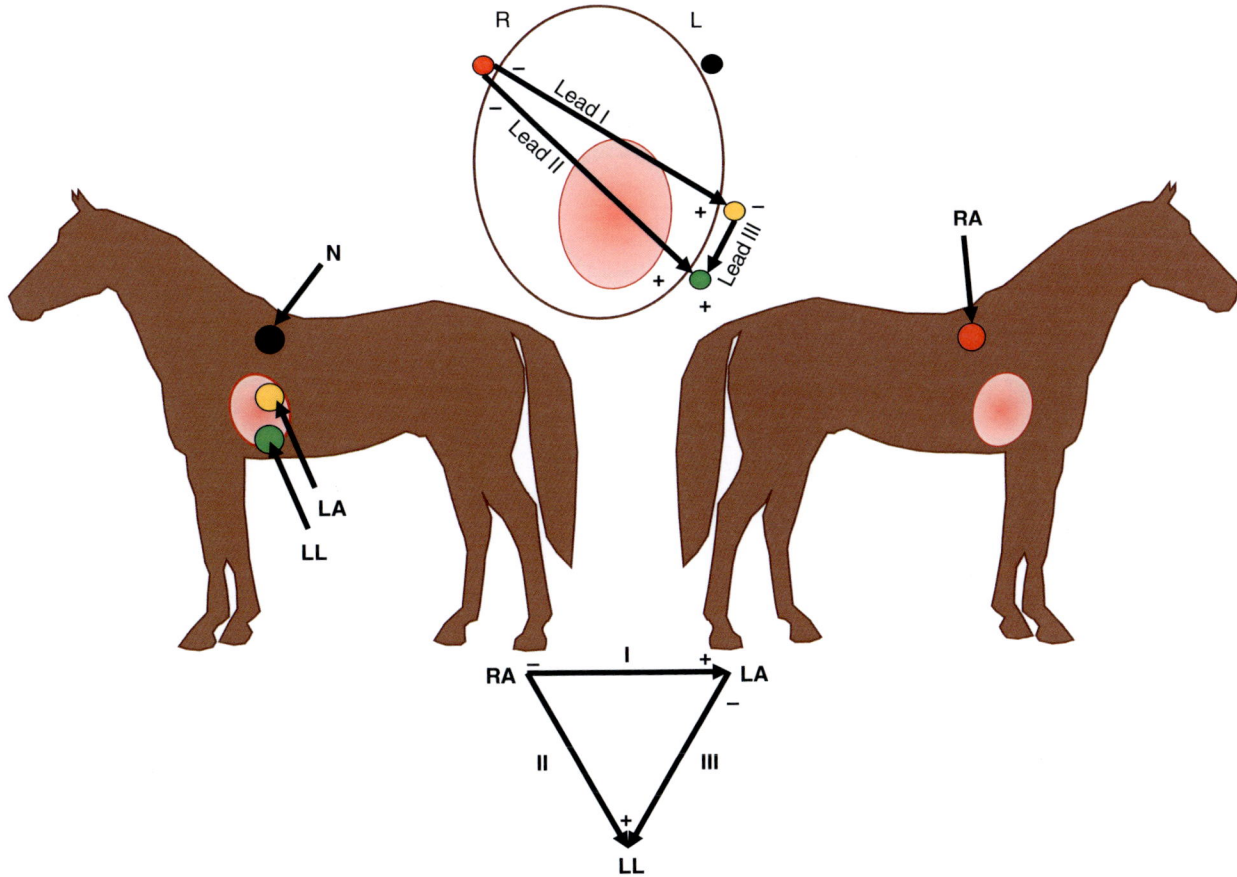

Fig. 2.2.

(A)

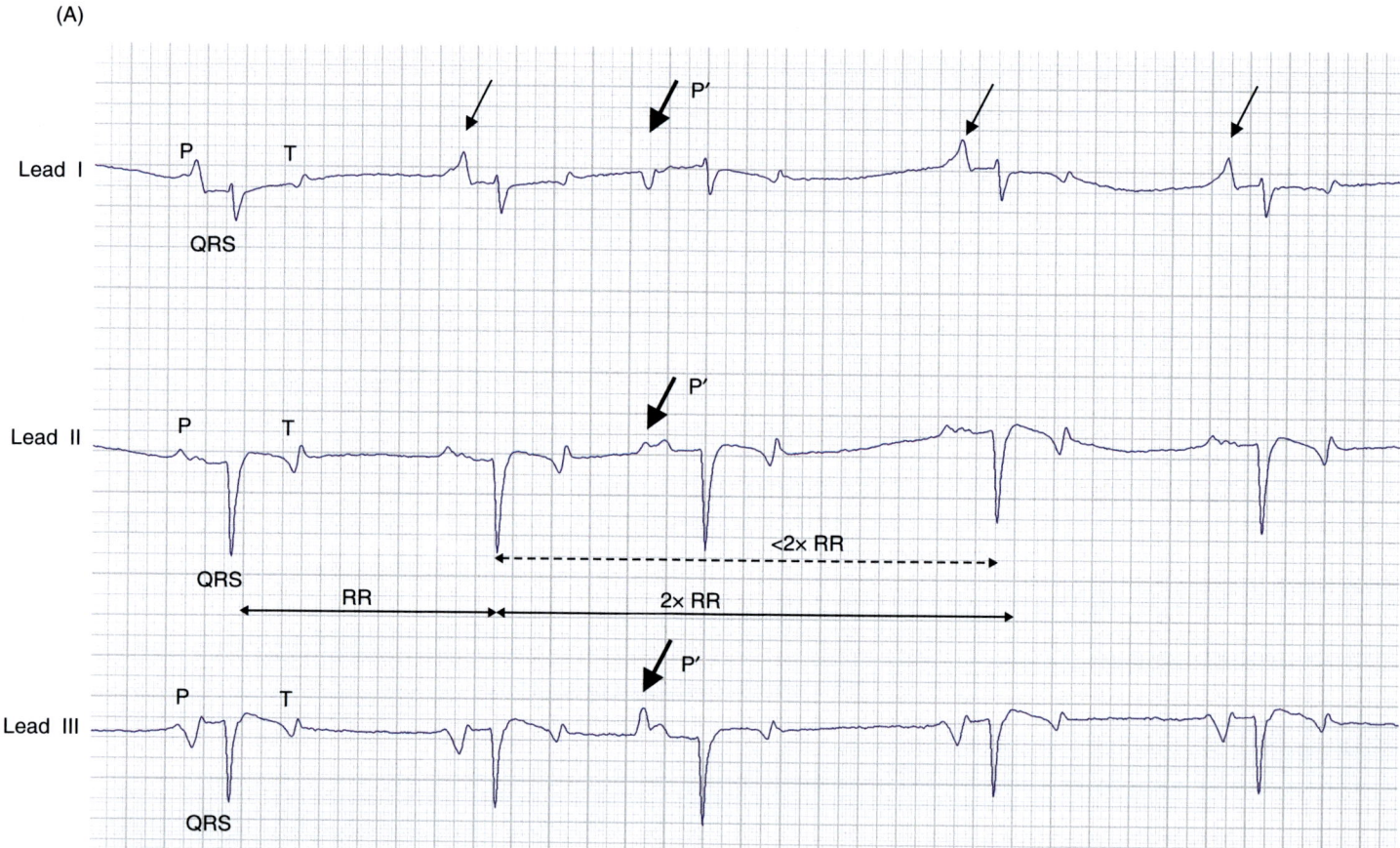

Fig. 2.3. See caption page 20.

(B)

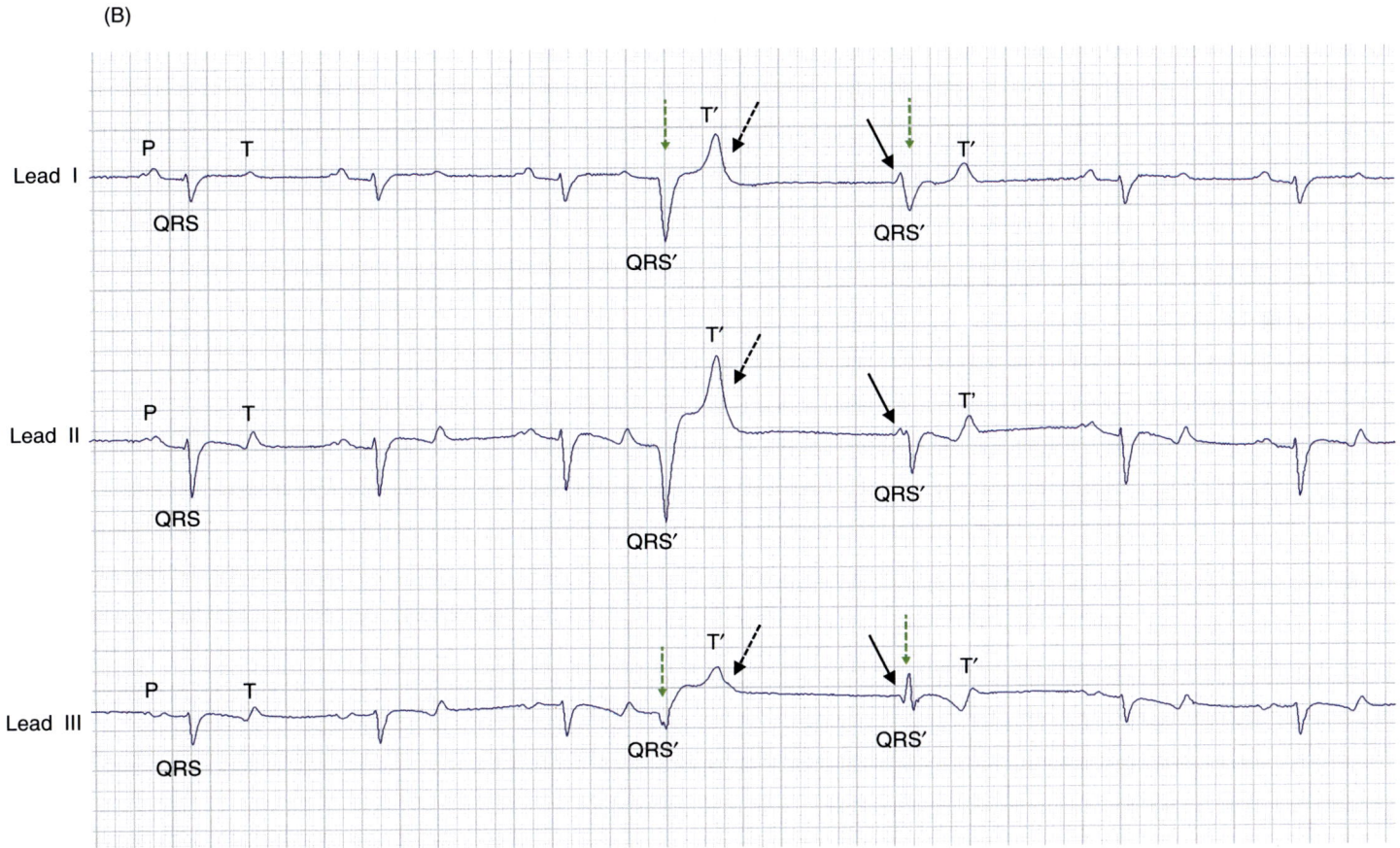

Fig. 2.3. Continued.

Longer-duration recordings

Recording an ECG for a longer period of time, particularly overnight or for 24 h, is useful for assessing the type, frequency and distribution of arrhythmias that may be present intermittently.

Normal horses can have varying numbers of vagally mediated arrhythmias at rest (Eggensperger and Schwarzwald, 2017). In a recent study, small numbers (on average <3/h) of premature complexes of atrial origin were present in just under 45% of overnight ECG recordings performed in healthy horses, while even smaller numbers (on average <1 every 3 h) of ventricular premature complexes were present in 4.3% of the horses (Zuber *et al.*, 2019).

Horses with clinically relevant but intermittent arrhythmias often have a much higher frequency of premature complexes, including couplets, triplets and short runs of tachycardia, and can show multiple P′ or QRS-T morphologies or evidence of a short coupling interval with the R-on-T phenomenon (superimposition of an ectopic beat on the T wave of a preceding beat), particularly at higher heart rates.

Fig. 2.3. Continued.
(A) An example of an ECG, recorded using the modified base–apex lead configuration described in Fig. 2.2. Lead I (RA→LA) provides useful information about the morphology of atrial premature complexes (P′, bold arrow), as the P (black arrows) and P′ waves are more prominent. One example of P′ morphology is depicted. Lead II (RA→LL) will produce the typical ECG. Lead III (LA→LL) will produce an alternative configuration, which can also aid in the detection of ectopic complexes (P′, bold arrow). In addition, the change in sinus rhythm following the atrial premature complex can be observed, with the sinoatrial node being depolarized ('reset'), slightly delaying the subsequent P wave. This results in the encompassing RR intervals (dashed double ended arrow) being less than twice the normal RR interval (solid double ended arrow). Paper speed: 50 mm/s. (B) An example of an ECG, recorded using the modified base–apex lead configuration described in Fig. 2.2. Lead I (RA→LA) provides useful information about the morphology of ventricular premature complexes (VPCs; dashed green arrows). Two different VPC morphologies are present. Lead II (RA→LL) will produce the typical ECG. Lead III (LA→LL) will produce an alternative configuration, which can also aid in the detection of ectopic complexes (green dashed arrows). Here, the underlying sinus rhythm is not interrupted, and P waves originating from the sinoatrial node can be seen buried in the T wave (black dashed arrow) and QRS complex (black arrow) of the abnormal ventricular complexes. Paper speed: 50 mm/s. RR, RR interval; 2× RR, twice the normal RR interval; <2× RR, less than twice the normal RR interval; P′, atrial premature complex P wave; QRS′, ventricular premature complex QRS wave; T′, premature complex T wave.

Bradyarrhythmias can also become apparent in longer recordings, especially overnight when the horse is not stimulated. Details on the identification and interpretation of specific arrhythmias in horses are discussed further in Chapters 3 and 4.

Extended ECG recordings coupled with video monitoring can be useful when investigating horses that present with collapse or weakness. Both recordings can be analysed simultaneously if any events occur during the period of observation. Implantable loop recorders for extended event monitoring should be considered in these cases, if the budget allows.

Table 2.1. Criteria for determining the duration of ECG recordings.

Indications for short-term recordings	Indications for long-term recordings (12–24 h)
Arrhythmia heard consistently during examination	History of arrhythmia but currently not apparent on auscultation
Screening to confirm normal sinus rhythm is present	Arrhythmia heard inconsistently during examination
Persistent tachyarrhythmia or bradyarrhythmia heard during examination	Horses with a history of weakness or collapse
	Monitoring response to therapy (e.g. anti-arrhythmics, heart-failure treatment)
	Monitoring of critically ill patients
	Horses with evidence of structural heart disease

Fig. 2.4. Continued.

Positioning of the ECG electrodes to obtain a modified base–apex recording from an exercising horse. (A, B) This electrode configuration (same as in Fig. 2.2) allows the three leads to each highlight different aspects of cardiac depolarization/repolarization (see Fig. 2.5A). This may not be practical for some exercise tests, particularly when a rider or equipment interferes with the electrode contact, creating artefacts. (C) This electrode configuration is useful for ridden exercise or when motion artefacts caused by equipment are present. The drawback of this placement is that both lead I (RA→LA) and lead II (RA→LL) are very similar, making abnormal morphology of complexes harder to detect (see Fig. 2.5B). RA, right arm electrode; LA, left arm electrode; LL, left leg (foot) electrode. Note that the colour system displayed here corresponds to the IEC standard (International Electrotechnical Commission) and is the one used by the Televet 100 recording system; other devices may use a different colour system (i.e. the one defined by the American Heart Association, where RA is white, LA is black, N is green and LL is red).

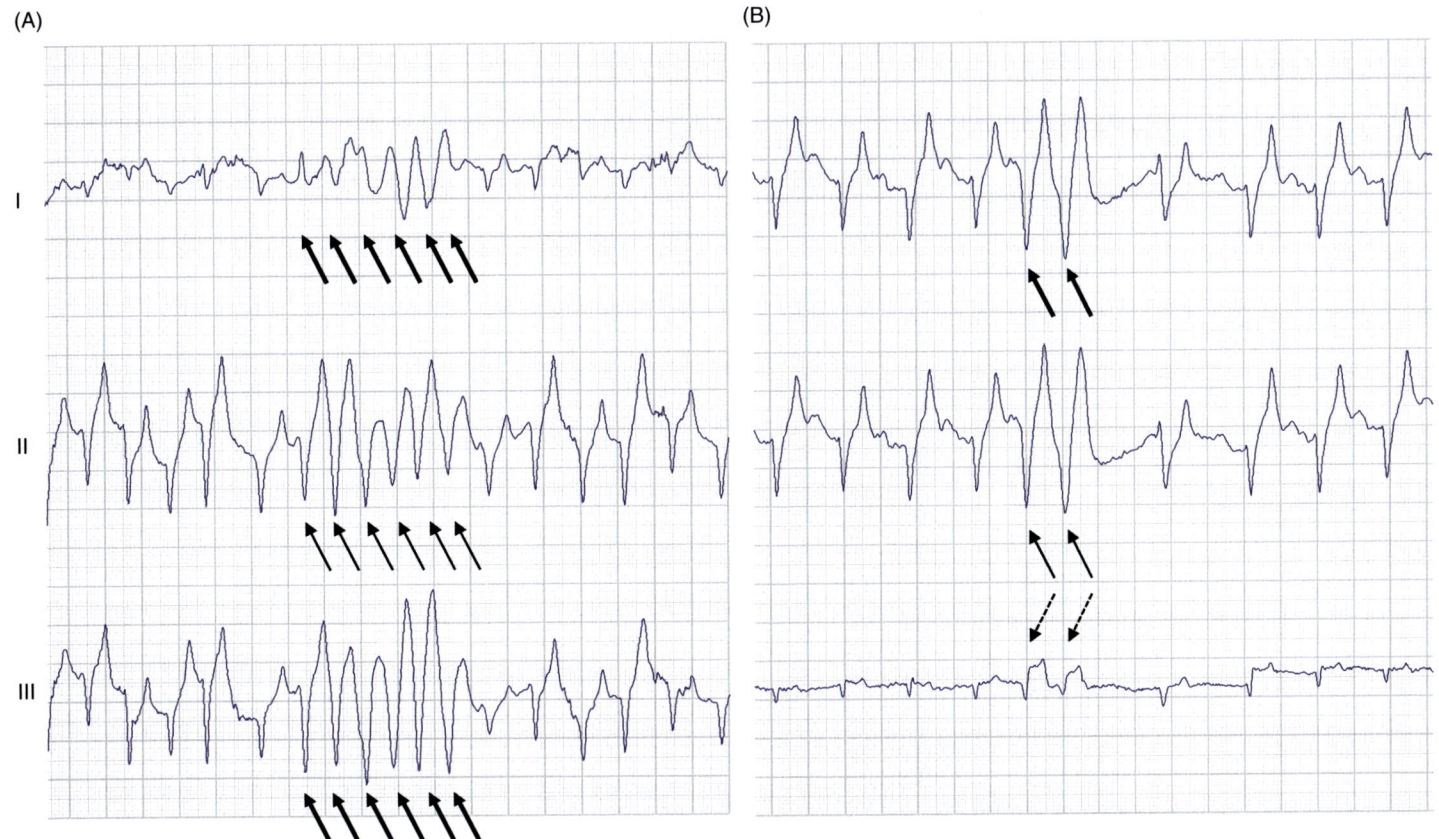

Fig. 2.5. See caption page 24.

Continuous mobile (ambulatory) ECG monitoring, in combination with telemetric live monitoring of the ECG signal, is frequently used to monitor the effectiveness of anti-arrhythmic or heart-failure therapy, or for observing trends in patients that are critically ill. In human and small-animal patients with heart disease, these extended ECG recordings are regularly repeated to provide diagnostic and prognostic information. This approach is also utilized in equine cardiology, although less supporting evidence for interpretation of any findings is currently available in the equine cardiology literature.

Exercising ECG Recording

The indications for performing an exercising ECG are provided in Box 2.2.

In horses with arrhythmias at rest, it can be informative to know whether the arrhythmia is 'overdrive suppressed' by the normal sinus rhythm at higher heart rates or whether additional arrhythmias develop (as seen, for example, in horses with atrial fibrillation that can develop wide-complex arrhythmias with a rapid ventricular response rate and R-on-T phenomenon during exercise or stress, as seen in Fig. 2.5A (Verheyen *et al.*, 2013).

When assessing for the presence of clinically relevant exercising arrhythmias, it is recommended that horses perform at or slightly above their intended level of exercise intensity. It is also important that the type of exercise is similar to the horse's typical work. Recording with a telemetric device allows continuous real-time assessment of the heart rate and rhythm both during and immediately after exercise,

Fig. 2.5. Continued.
(A) An example of an ECG recorded using the modified base–apex lead configuration described in Fig. 2.4A and B. This is an exercising ECG performed in a horse with atrial fibrillation and a period of rapid ventricular conduction with R-on-T phenomenon is present. Lead I and lead III provide useful information about the morphology of abnormal QRS-T waves (bold arrows) that was not as apparent in the lead II recording (thin arrows). (B) An example of an ECG recorded using the modified base–apex lead configuration described in Fig. 2.4C. Both lead I (RA→LA) and lead II (RA→LL) are similar, which provides a back-up lead in case one is dislodged during exercise. However, abnormal morphology is not as easy to detect as with the electrode configuration seen in Fig. 2.4A and B. A couplet of ventricular premature complexes (lead I, bold arrows; lead II, thin arrows; lead III, dotted arrows) are shown. Paper speed: 50 mm/s.

Box 2.2. Indications for performing an exercising ECG.

- A history of exercise intolerance or poor performance.
- A history of weakness or collapse.
- Horses with evidence of structural heart disease.
- Horses with atrial fibrillation, to determine the heart rate during exercise and screen for other concurrent arrhythmias.
- Horses with frequent arrhythmias at rest.
- Horses where an arrhythmia was detected during recovery after exercise.

where arrhythmias are most commonly observed. This allows the exercise test to be terminated if pathological rhythms or exceedingly high heart rates are detected. It is also important to analyse thoroughly the exercising ECG after the test has been concluded, as subtle abnormalities may only be visible with detailed page-by-page evaluation of the rhythm (see Chapter 3).

It can be technically challenging to record good-quality exercising ECG recordings. Careful preparation is key, paying particular attention to the placement of the electrodes to avoid motion artefacts associated with equipment or rider movement. The use of adhesive material covering any electrodes or cables can provide additional stability (Fig. 2.1A). Several tested devices include built-in electrodes to avoid the problem of dislodgement during strenuous exercise, although these devices are not readily available.

Optimization of the ECG recording quality is of utmost importance, as the detection of arrhythmias during periods of high heart rate, where motion artefacts are also present, can be very difficult. Examples of motion artefacts during exercise are seen in Fig. 2.6. If necessary, the exercise test should be interrupted and the electrode positioning adjusted, in order to obtain a diagnostic-quality ECG recording. In addition, differentiating between normal variation and pathological arrhythmias can be difficult, although recent studies suggest that there is very little normal beat-to-beat variation present during peak exercise in healthy horses (Fig. 2.7) (Frick *et al.*, 2019; Flethoj *et al.*, 2016).

The use of ECGs to assess the heart rate and rhythm in horses during exercise is far more widespread than the use of longer-duration resting recordings, and a larger body of evidence is available in the literature characterizing the normal and abnormal findings in exercising horses. This is covered extensively in Chapters 3, 4 and 6.

Tips for Obtaining Good-quality Recordings

Recording good-quality diagnostic ECGs is essential, regardless of whether the ECG is recorded for 2 min, 24 h or during exercise. Careful attention should be given to the placement of electrodes, ensuring adequate contact with the skin surface for optimal conduction of the electrical signal. The use of additional adhesive material (Fig. 2.1A) on top of the gel electrode/cable unit can improve

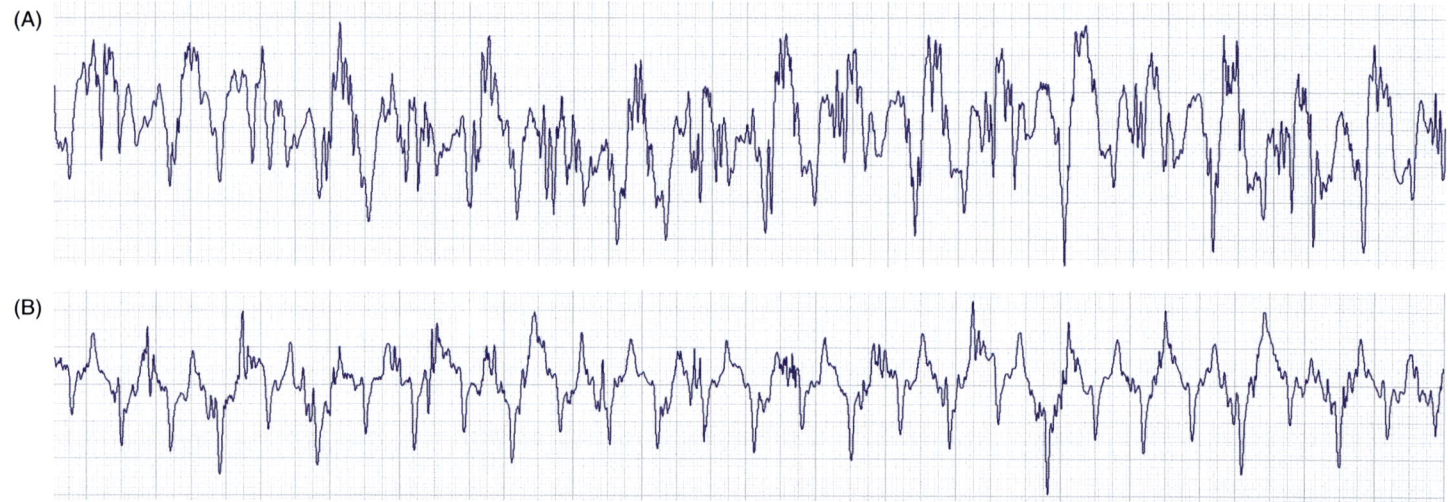

Fig. 2.6. (A) A non-diagnostic-quality exercising ECG trace, where frequent motion artefacts interfere with the quality of the ECG recording and make it difficult to identify the normal QRS complexes. Paper speed 50 mm/s. (B) A poor-quality exercising ECG trace, where frequent motion artefacts obscure the baseline, but QRS complexes can be regularly detected. Some QRS complexes appear wider, rounded or fragmented as a result of these artefacts, which will interfere with subsequent RR interval analysis. Paper speed 50 mm/s.

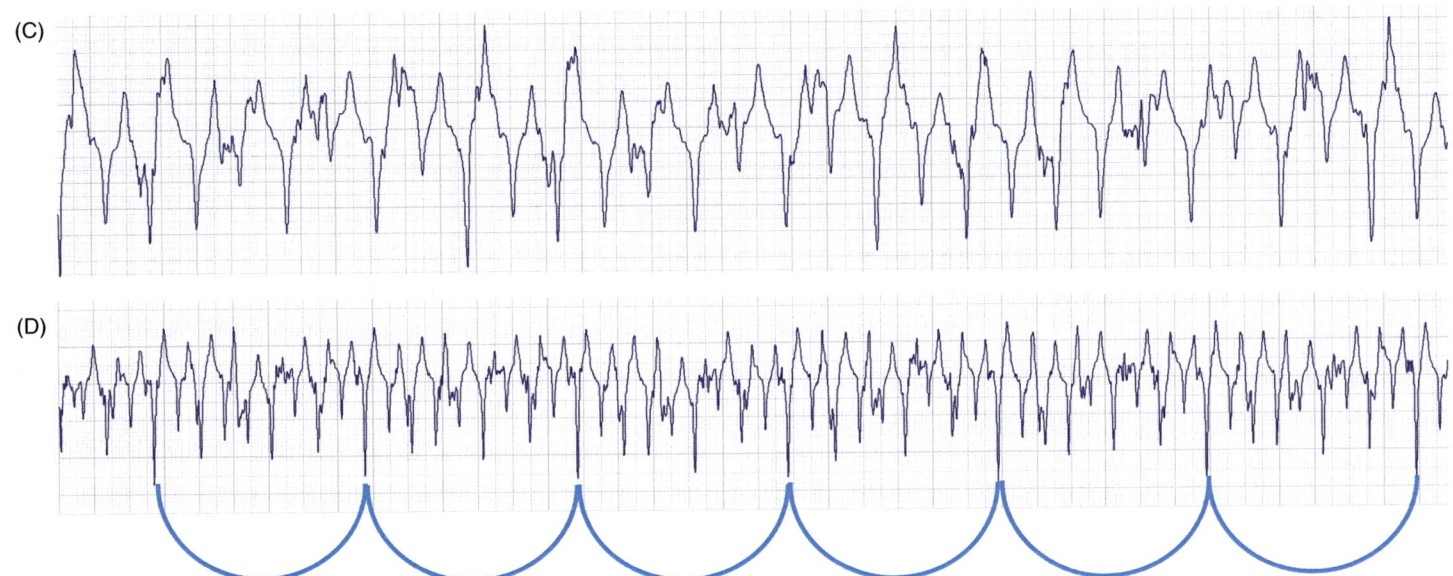

Fig. 2.6. Continued.

(C) A good-quality exercising ECG recording. Motion artefacts are still observed but do not interfere with the QRS morphology and the ability to perform RR interval analysis. Paper speed 50 mm/s. (D) An overview of an exercising ECG recording where repetitive motion artefacts can be observed. These motion artefacts appear to be coupled with stride or respiratory frequency. These recurrent artefacts result in larger-appearing QRS complexes (blue half circles), which should not be interpreted as abnormal. Paper speed 25 mm/s.

(A)

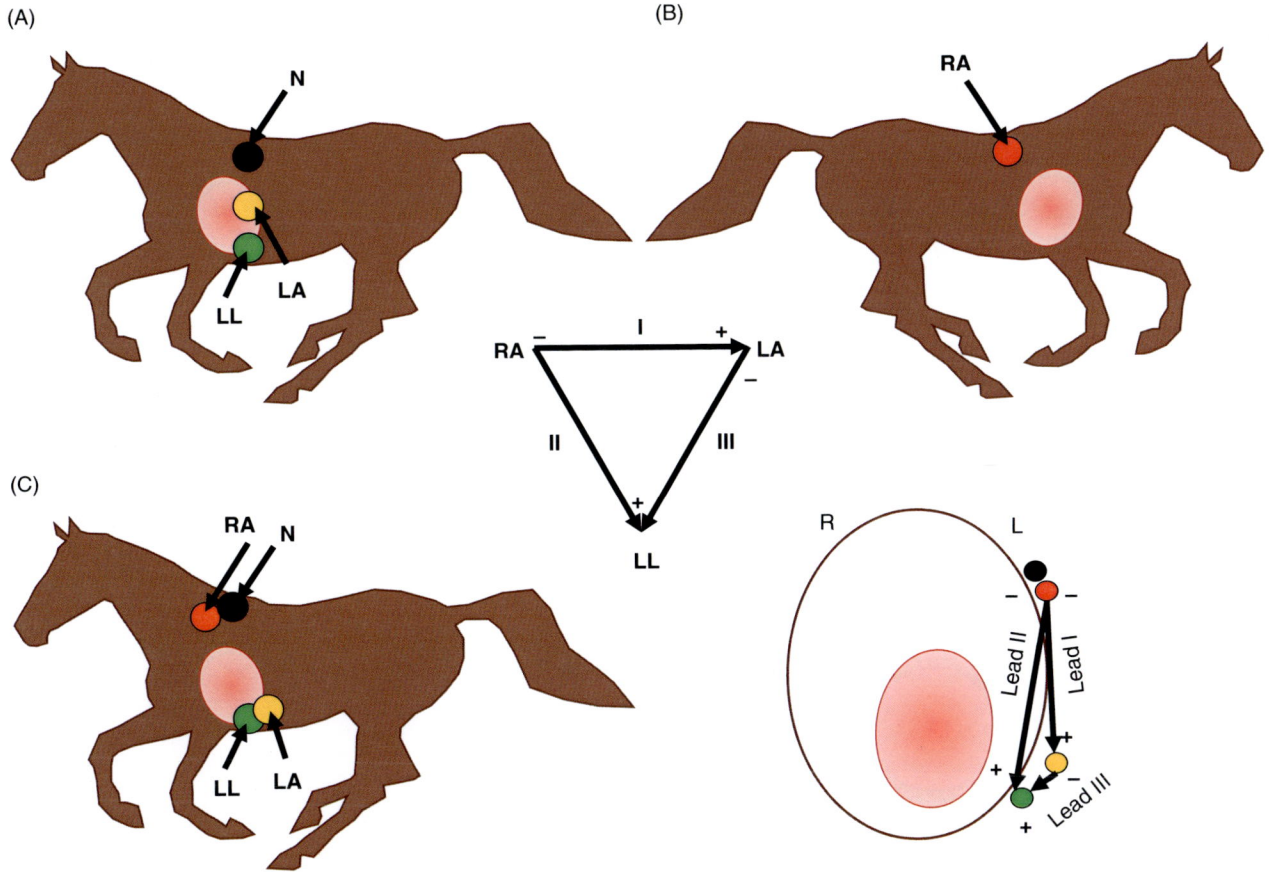

(B)

(C)

Fig. 2.4. See caption page 22.

the robustness of the contact, particularly for extended-duration recordings or situations where electrode contact may be disrupted (e.g. sweating during exercise).

Regular monitoring of the ECG recording quality is also important, so that any problems (e.g. electrodes coming off, batteries exhausted) can be identified and quickly rectified without interfering with the duration of the diagnostic recording. When the ECG quality is suboptimal, steps should be taken to problem solve the issue by checking the placement and contact of the electrodes (and replacing them where necessary); the placement of the cables, surcingle and recording device; and the connections between the electrodes, cables and recording device.

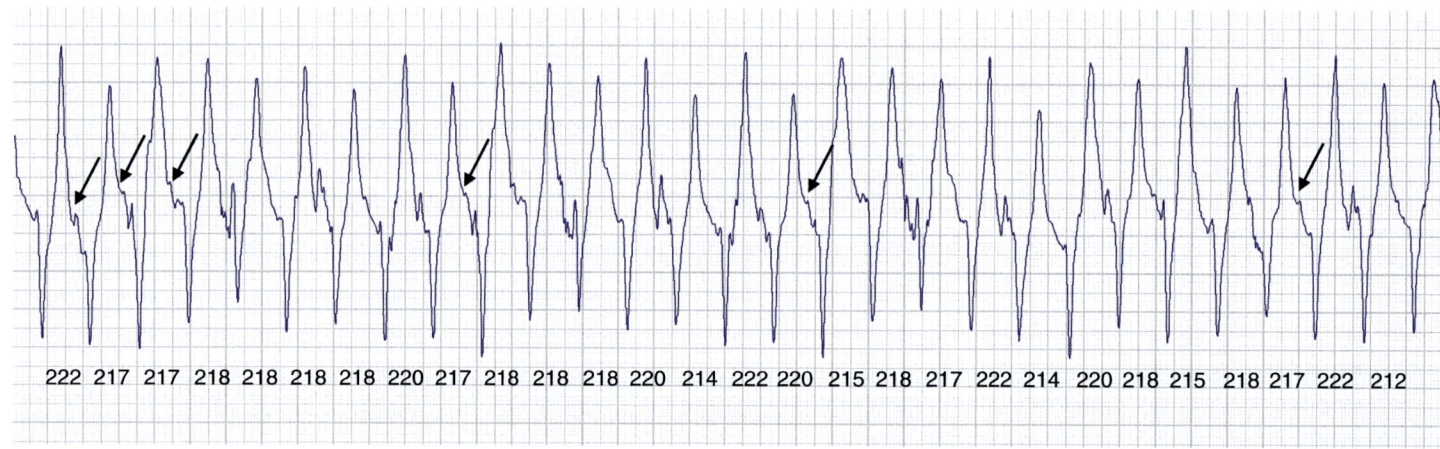

Fig. 2.7. An excellent-quality exercising ECG recording. The QRS complexes are easily identified and a lack of motion artefacts allows occasional P waves (black arrows) also to be identified. The instantaneous heart rate is displayed below (bpm) showing very little beat-to-beat variation between consecutive complexes. Paper speed: 50 mm/s.

Analysing ECGs

Overview and Basic Rhythm Analysis

When evaluating an ECG, it is recommended to use a systematic, logical approach, which ensures that all useful information is gathered from the recording. This process is described in Table 3.1 and includes information about heart rate, rhythm and waveform morphology. As most equine ECGs are recorded using a 'base–apex' or 'modified base–apex' three-lead configuration, as opposed to the 12-lead ECGs recording from human patients or small animals, calculation of the mean electrical axis is not a routine part of the equine ECG evaluation.

It is also critical to be familiar with the normal equine P-QRS-T morphology (see Fig. 1.3, Chapter 1) and the appearance of artefacts (Box 3.1 and Fig. 3.1) and commonly-occurring physiological arrhythmias (described in Chapter 4).

Detailed Rhythm Analysis

Short-duration ECGs (2–5 min) can be analysed quickly with visual inspection in most cases. Exercising ECGs or longer-term resting recordings can be time-consuming to analyse in detail.

For this, we also follow a logical staged approach, as detailed in Table 3.2 (Frick *et al.*, 2019; Mitchell, 2019).

Table 3.1. Basic ECG analysis: a stepwise approach.

Step 1	First, the overall quality of the recording is assessed:
	• The P-QRS-T complexes should be clearly visible and free of obvious artefacts (see Box 3.1 and Fig. 3.1).
	• Do not perform a detailed analysis if the recording quality is poor/non-diagnostic, as misdiagnosis of the rhythm is possible.
Step 2	Identify the paper speed (typically 25 or 50 mm/s) and calculate the overall heart rate.
	• Compare the heart rate with the reported reference ranges, as these are body-weight dependent (Schwarzwald *et al.*, 2012).
	• The heart rate can be divided into three broad categories: normal, bradycardic or tachycardic.
	• Many digital systems will perform automated RR interval analysis and then calculate and display the instantaneous heart rate.
	• If the rhythm is irregular, a longer period of ECG should be used to assess the heart rate and a heart-rate range can be reported.
Step 3	Assess whether the rhythm is regular or irregular:
	• If the rhythm is irregular, is there any underlying pattern (regularly irregular) or is there no pattern (irregularly irregular)?
	• Are there pauses, premature complexes or both? Are they related to one another (i.e. a premature complex followed by a pause)?
	• If there are pauses, how long are the pauses (shorter than twice the normal RR, twice the normal RR or longer than twice the normal RR)?
	• If there are premature complexes, it can be helpful to measure the RR intervals encompassing the abnormal beat (i.e. for one abnormal beat, measure 2× the normal RR; for two abnormal beats, measure 3× the normal RR, etc., and then trace the preceding and the subsequent R waves to determine whether the underlying sinus rhythm is disrupted or not). Examples are given in Chapter 4 and shown in Figs 2.3A and 3.2.
Step 4	Identify the most normal-appearing P-QRS-T complexes (if present) and then compare them with the abnormal complexes. For every complex ask:
	• Is there a P for every QRS?
	• Is there a QRS for every P?
	• If no clear P waves are identified – can flutter (F) or fibrillation (f) waves be seen? Examples shown in Fig. 4.12 and 4.14.
	• Do P and QRS complexes appear related (similar PR intervals) or dissociated (varying PR intervals, P waves 'wandering' in and out of the QRS complexes)?
	• Is the morphology of all P-QRS-T complexes similar or does morphology vary? Examples are shown in Fig. 3.3.
	• In particular, are all T waves the same or is there variation in T-wave morphology that could be caused by secondary T-wave changes (i.e. if the preceding QRS is abnormal, then the following T wave is likely to be abnormal as well) or superimposition of other waves (e.g. a P′ wave within the preceding T wave)? Examples are shown in Fig. 3.3.

Continued

Table 3.1. Continued.

Step 5	Measure the PR, QRS and QT intervals: • Are they similar or varying? • Compare the intervals with the reference ranges, as these are body-weight and heart-rate dependent (Schwarzwald *et al.*, 2012).
Step 6	Define the rhythm: • Is this a disorder of abnormal impulse formation, abnormal impulse conduction or both? • Is the rhythm primarily sinus in origin? If not, are the abnormal complexes of atrial, junctional or ventricular origin? • Is the rhythm sustained or paroxysmal? • What is the timing and frequency of occurrence of abnormal beats?
Step 7	If unsure about the rhythm diagnosis or interpretation of the clinical relevance, seek a second opinion from a person experienced in equine ECG interpretation.

Box 3.1. Criteria for recognizing artefacts.

• Look for normal QRS complexes at regular intervals within the tracing.
• Every QRS *must* be followed by a T wave; artefacts do not have T waves.
• The normal QRS complex represents the fastest conduction pathway, all *abnormal* QRS complexes must be *wider* (and therefore slower) than the normal QRS complexes. Artefacts are frequently narrower than the normal QRS complexes.
• Check the other lead recordings – artefacts can be less obvious in other leads while real findings should be present in all leads.

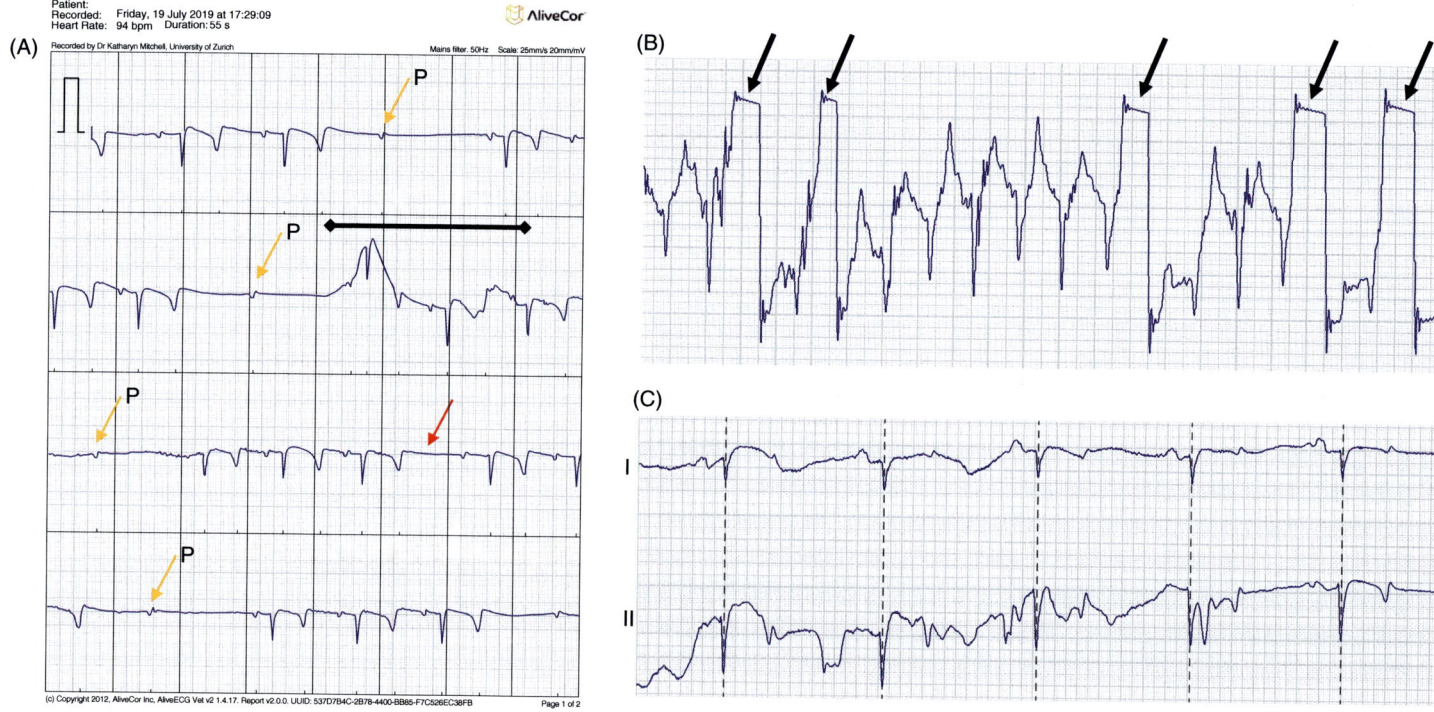

Fig. 3.1. See caption page 33

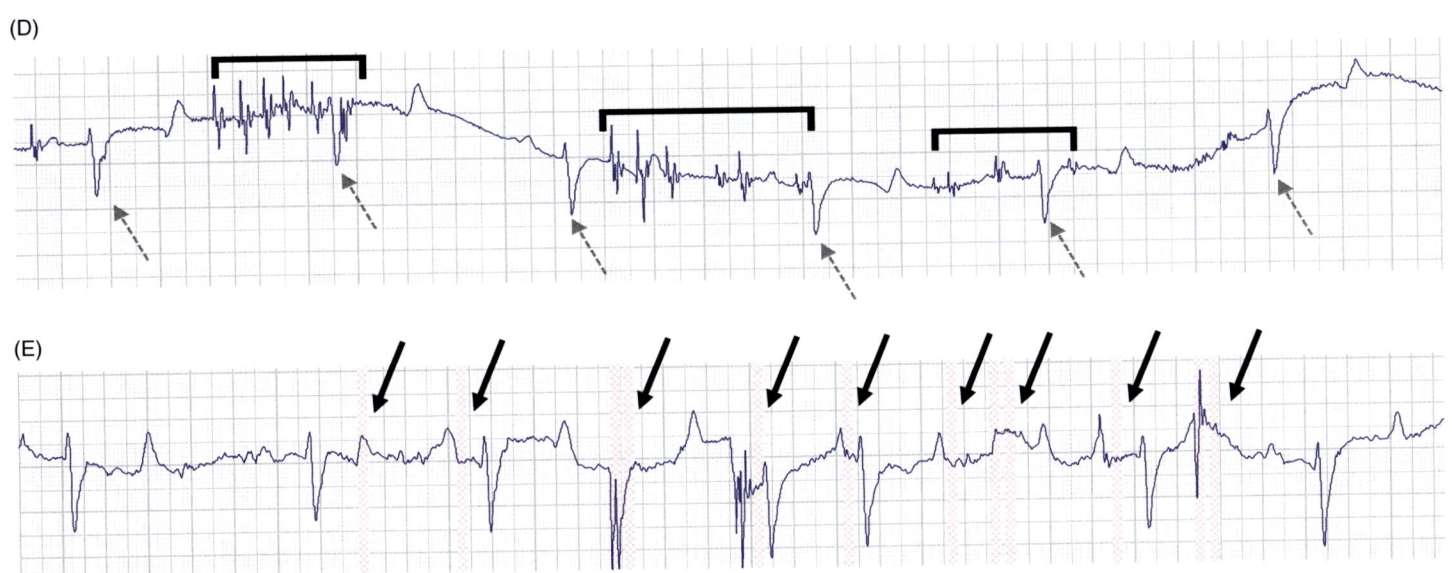

Fig. 3.1. Examples of artefacts that interfere with ECG interpretation. (A) A short-duration ECG recorded with a hand-held device (AliveCor KardiaMobile ECG; Alivecor, Mountain View, California, USA). Note the poorly-diagnostic section of the ECG (double-ended black line), where P-QRS-T morphology is not clearly differentiated from the motion artefacts. In addition, there is a sinus arrhythmia with a sinus pause (red arrow) and second-degree atrioventricular blocks (yellow arrows). (B) An exercising ECG with frequent artefacts (bold arrows) caused by a broken cable with exposed wiring. (C) Frequent motion artefacts are present along the baseline of the ECG recording; however, regular QRS complexes can still be identified (grey dashed lines) particularly in lead I. (D) Frequent skin-twitching motion artefacts and baseline wander (black bars); however, regular QRS complexes can still be identified (grey dashed arrows). (E) Red hashed lines (bold arrows) indicate poor Bluetooth connectivity, causing interruption in the sending of the digitalized ECG recording to the monitor. This problem can be avoided by recording the ECG directly (i.e. on to an SD card) in addition to transmitting the signal wirelessly and performing any additional analyses on the directly recorded ECG.

Table 3.2. Detailed, advanced ECG analysis: a stepwise approach.

Step 1	Assess ECG recording quality:
	• Non-diagnostic-quality ECGs (where P-QRS-T morphology cannot be clearly determined for long periods) should not be analysed.
Step 2	Screen for obvious rhythm events:
	• This can be done using an 'overview' screen, which many of the software systems provide.
	• Changes to QRS-T morphology and heart rate can often easily be detected with the level of detail present on an overview screen, with the relevant segments of the ECG then 'zoomed' in for further examination.
Step 3	Perform RR interval analysis:
	• Depending on the software program, this is an automated feature.
	• Software detects the R wave of the QRS complex, and then calculates the RR interval and instantaneous heart rate.
	• Some software allows for manual override of the QRS detection, which allows errors in detection to be corrected.
	• Some software will apply an 'alert' (i.e. different colour) when an RR interval is shorter or longer than a predetermined limit. This can be helpful when screening for premature complexes or pauses; however, there are many limitations to this technique, and complexes with normal timing but abnormal morphology may be overlooked.
Step 4	Morphology analysis:
	• Some software programs (particularly the human or small-animal Holter software programs) will utilize algorithms that detect variations in morphology of the P-QRS-T complexes.
	• These programs can be time-consuming to use for equine ECG evaluation due to the frequent variation in P and T morphology that is seen with increasing or decreasing heart rate. This variation can be normal in horses but will be detected as abnormal by the software algorithms. Therefore, these programs require manual verification of the morphology classifications.
	• If automated morphology analysis is not available, manual morphology analysis can be performed with 'full disclosure', i.e. page-by-page analysis of the ECG or utilizing the overview screen to detect obvious changes in morphology.
Step 5	Graphical analysis:
	• A useful way to examine exercising ECGs or longer-duration resting ECG data can be through graphical analysis.
	• Export of corrected, sequential RR intervals is possible from some ECG software programs, while the human and small-animal ECG software programs often provide graphical analysis automatically.
	• The most simple and useful are the heart-rate time-series tachogram, RR interval time-series tachogram and Poincaré graphs.
	• These graphs can be created in readily available software programs such as Excel, GraphPad Prism or Kubios HRV software.

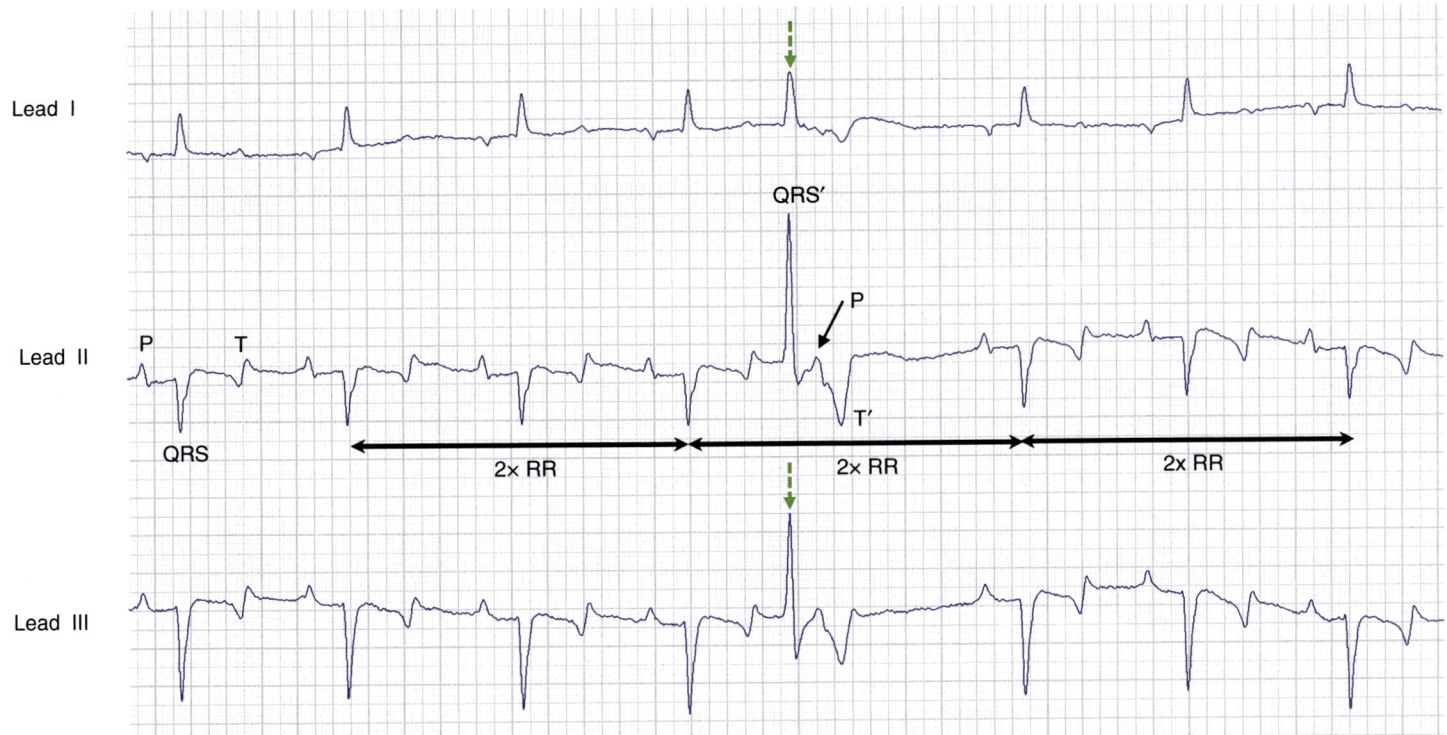

Fig. 3.2. An example of an ECG, recorded using the modified base–apex lead configuration described in Fig. 2.2. A ventricular prema-ture complex (green dashed arrow) is present. The QRS′ morphology is completely different (Rs rather than S) and the abnormal QRS′ complex is much wider than the normal QRS. Here, the underlying sinus rhythm is not interrupted (due to the atrioventricular node blocking retrograde conduction to the atria). A normal P wave originating from the sinoatrial node can be seen buried in the ST segment (black arrow) of the abnormal ventricular complex. As a result of the premature depolarization, the ventricular tissue is refractory and the sinus beat is not conducted. This pause results in the encompassing RR intervals being twice the normal RR interval (2×RR, double-ended arrows). Paper speed: 50 mm/s. QRS′, ventricular premature complex QRS; T′, premature complex T wave.

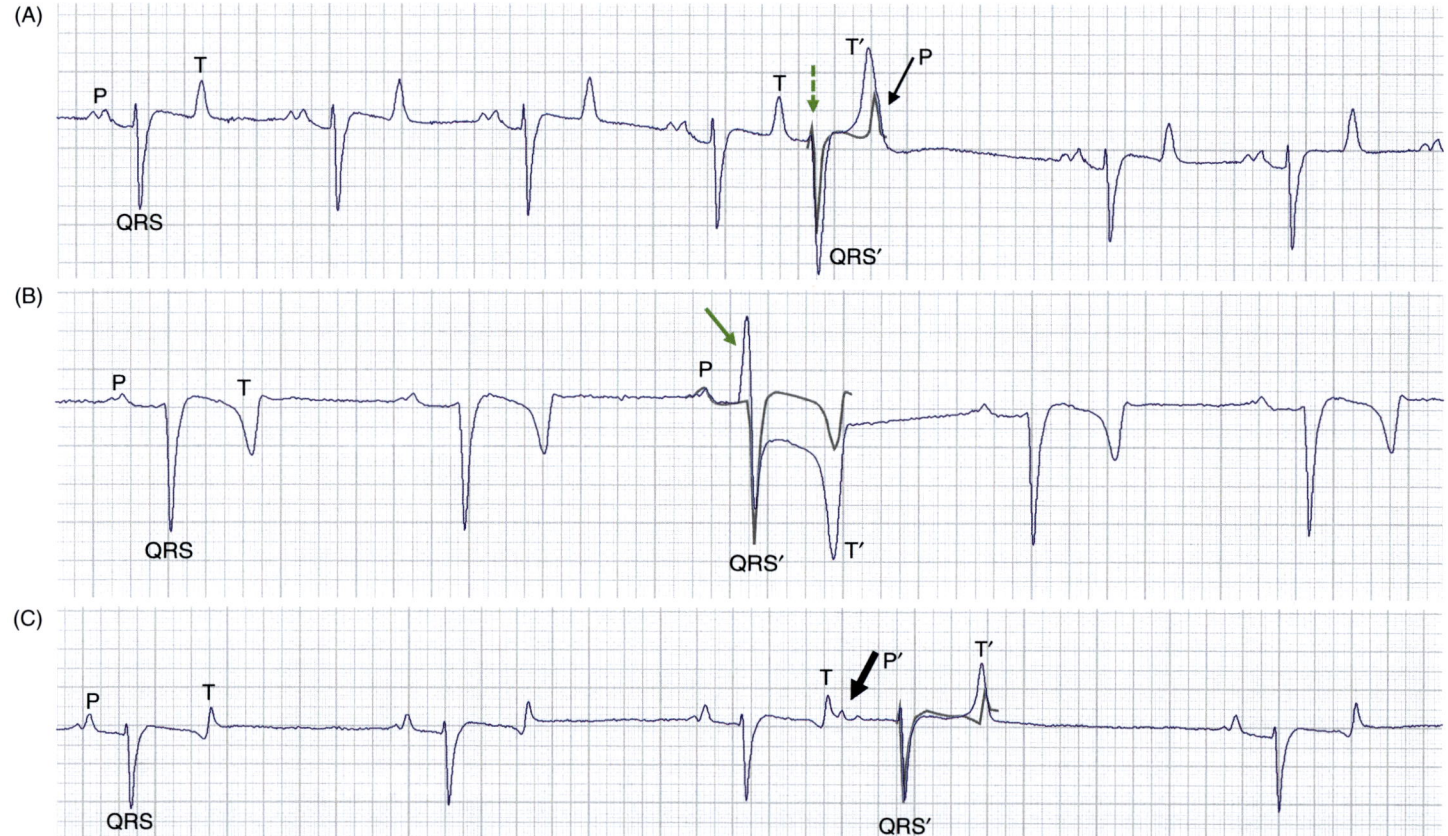

Fig. 3.3. See caption page 37

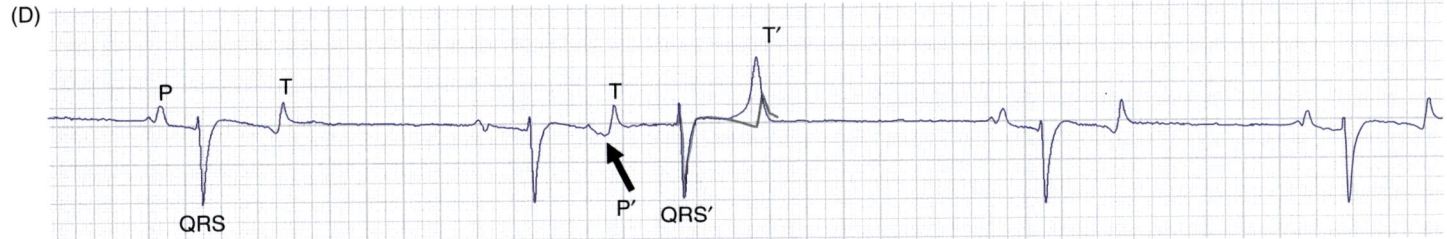

Fig. 3.3. Examples of different QRS-T morphologies. (A) A ventricular premature complex is present (green dashed arrow). The normal QRS morphology (grey) is superimposed over the abnormal complex. The abnormal complex is clearly wider and larger than the normal morphology, while the T wave is much larger. A normal P wave (black arrow) is buried in the abnormal T wave, and is not conducted, resulting in a pause after the premature complex. (B) A fusion complex is present (green solid arrow). This is where, due to the timing (long coupling interval) of the premature complex, a normal QRS complex (superimposed in grey) is fused with an abnormal ventricular complex. A normal P wave is present, and then the premature QRS complex results in a shorter PQ interval. The QRS′ starts with an abnormal positive wave (R) and finishes with the normal S wave. The T wave of the fusion beat is much larger but of similar polarity to that of the normal complexes. There is no change in the underlying sinus rhythm. (C) An atrial premature complex is present. The premature P wave is present (P′, bold arrow) with different morphology to the normal P waves. The premature complex has a normal QRS morphology (normal superimposed in grey) but there are secondary T-wave changes present, most likely because of the short coupling interval of the premature complex to the preceding beat. Because the atrial premature complex has also depolarized the sinoatrial (SA) node, there is a pause in the sinus rhythm (SA node reset) after the premature complex. (D) An atrial premature complex is present. The premature P wave is present (P′, bold arrow) buried in the ST segment of the preceding complex and has a different morphology to the normal P waves. The premature complex has a subtly different QRS morphology (normal superimposed in grey) with a larger r wave and deeper S wave and there are secondary T-wave changes present, most likely because of the short coupling interval of the premature complex to the preceding beat. Because the atrial premature complex also depolarized the SA node, there is a pause in the sinus rhythm (SA node reset) after the premature complex. Paper speed: 50 mm/s.

Heart-Rate Variability Analysis

Heart-rate variability (HRV) is the term used to describe oscillations in rate between consecutive cardiac cycles. Indices of variability can be calculated using either instantaneous heart-rate or RR interval data, exported from the ECG software. The traditional use of HRV in human medicine has centred around investigating autonomic balance (sympathetic and parasympathetic inputs) in healthy and diseased states. Standardized guidelines exist for the analysis and interpretation of HRV in human patients, but no such standardized guidelines exist for veterinary use (Task Force of the European Society of Cardiology/North American Society of Pacing Electrophysiology, 1996). This is problematic, as HRV analysis is performed regularly in veterinary medicine, but without a standardized approach to obtaining recordings, recording devices and analysis, the results of such studies are difficult to compare and utilize clinically. Factors to consider when wanting to perform HRV analysis are shown in Box 3.2.

HRV analysis can be divided into three main components of analysis: (i) time-domain analysis; (ii) frequency-domain analysis; and (iii) non-linear methods. Time-domain analysis is the simplest group of calculations to understand and can be further divided into statistical and graphical (i.e. Poincaré plots, histograms) methods of representation. Frequency-domain analysis involves various spectral methods of tachogram transformation to determine the total power and low-frequency and high-frequency components of HRV. Non-linear analysis is an evolving field in HRV and involves complex mathematical equations and transformation. From these three groups, the various HRV parameters can also be described as short-term components (high-frequency/vagal inputs), longer-term components (low-frequency/sympathetic inputs) or overall measures of HRV. The commonly calculated parameters are described in Table 3.3.

Traditional HRV analysis has been performed on longer-term ECG recordings, with abnormal complexes being deliberately excluded in the post-processing (often by using software filters). This allows the focus of any inherent variability in RR intervals to be attributed to sinoatrial node function and thus reflect the balance between the parasympathetic and sympathetic nervous system inputs into the sino-atrial node. The resulting RR sequence (without arrhythmias) is referred to as the normal–normal (NN) interval.

HRV analysis has been utilized in human medicine across a wide variety of fields, from detecting fetal distress to predicting heart failure following myocardial infarction or assessing the effect of overtraining in athletes (Malik *et al.*, 1996; Woo *et al.*, 1992; Dong, 2016).

Box 3.2. Factors to consider standardizing when collecting and analysing data for heart-rate variability analysis.

- Type of recording device (e.g. traditional ECG recording vs heart-rate monitor).
- Timing of the recording, as there is considerable fluctuation in HRV parameters over a 24 h period
- Length of recording: this is particularly important when looking at indices of long-term HRV.
- Use of RR interval or PP interval data sets in horses, given the frequent occurrence of second-degree atrioventricular blocks at rest in some horses.
- Resting versus exercising recordings.
- Post-processing, filtering and automated 'black box' analysis.

Table 3.3. Common terminology used in heart-rate variability analysis.

Analysis	Term	Definition
Overall HRV assessment	Mean heart rate	
	Mean RR (NN) interval	
	SDNN	Standard deviation of NN intervals
	Triangular index	Integral of NN interval histogram, divided by the height of the histogram
	TINN	Triangular interpolation of the NN interval histogram
	Total power	Variance of all NN intervals
	LF:HF	Ratio of low- to high-frequency power
Short-term components (high-frequency/vagal input)	RMSSD	Square root of mean squared differences between successive NN intervals
	SD1	Standard deviation of Poincaré plot, perpendicular to the line of identity (mathematically identical to RMSSD)
	HF	High-frequency spectral components
Long-term components (low-frequency/ sympathetic ± vagal inputs)	SDANN	Standard deviation of the average NN intervals in all non-overlapping 5 min segments
	SD2	Standard deviation of the Poincaré plot, along the line of identity
	LF	Low-frequency spectral components

NN, normal–normal.

HRV analysis in horses has been used for many applications to date. Some of these have been purely investigating physiological or pathophysiological mechanisms in a research setting, while others have been applied to clinical practice in an attempt to provide diagnostic and prognostic information. Frequently used applications include (but are certainly not limited to) cardiology and exercise physiology investigations, monitoring the response to stress, training or overtraining, outcomes following colic surgery, welfare evaluations and fetal viability monitoring (Thayer *et al.*, 1997; Rietmann *et al.*, 2004; Kinnunen *et al.*, 2006; Ohmura *et al.*, 2006; von Borell *et al.*, 2007; McConachie *et al.*, 2016; Broux *et al.*, 2017; Eggensperger and Schwarzwald, 2017; Heliczer *et al.*, 2017).

Interpretation of Arrhythmias

Decision-tree algorithms to aid in classifying arrhythmias are presented in Figs 4.1, 4.2 and 4.3. Correct identification of the arrhythmia is important for deciding on the most appropriate therapy, for advising on long-term prognosis and for the assessment of risk of an adverse event.

It is important to recognize physiological variations in rhythm that can be completely normal in horses, particularly at rest, but that, when occurring during exercise or at higher heart rates, can be considered pathological.

Physiological Arrhythmias

Many of the common physiological arrhythmias observed in horses are related to tonic vagal inhibition of the SA and AV nodal tissue. Therefore, they are frequently documented at rest and during changing autonomic balance (e.g. in the recovery phase after exercise, where sympathetic tone withdraws and parasympathetic tone increases). Examples of physiological rhythms are seen in Figs 4.4–4.6.

Sinus arrhythmia

Sinus arrhythmia is a common finding in horses at rest and after exercise (Fig. 4.4). The heart rate typically speeds up and slows down in a phasic manner. Unlike in small animals, these heart-rate changes are not usually associated with the respiratory cycle. Changes in P-wave morphology can result from a wandering pacemaker within the SA node, and this is a common finding in addition to sinus arrhythmia. The P waves can also become larger with increasing heart rate and smaller with slowing heart rate.

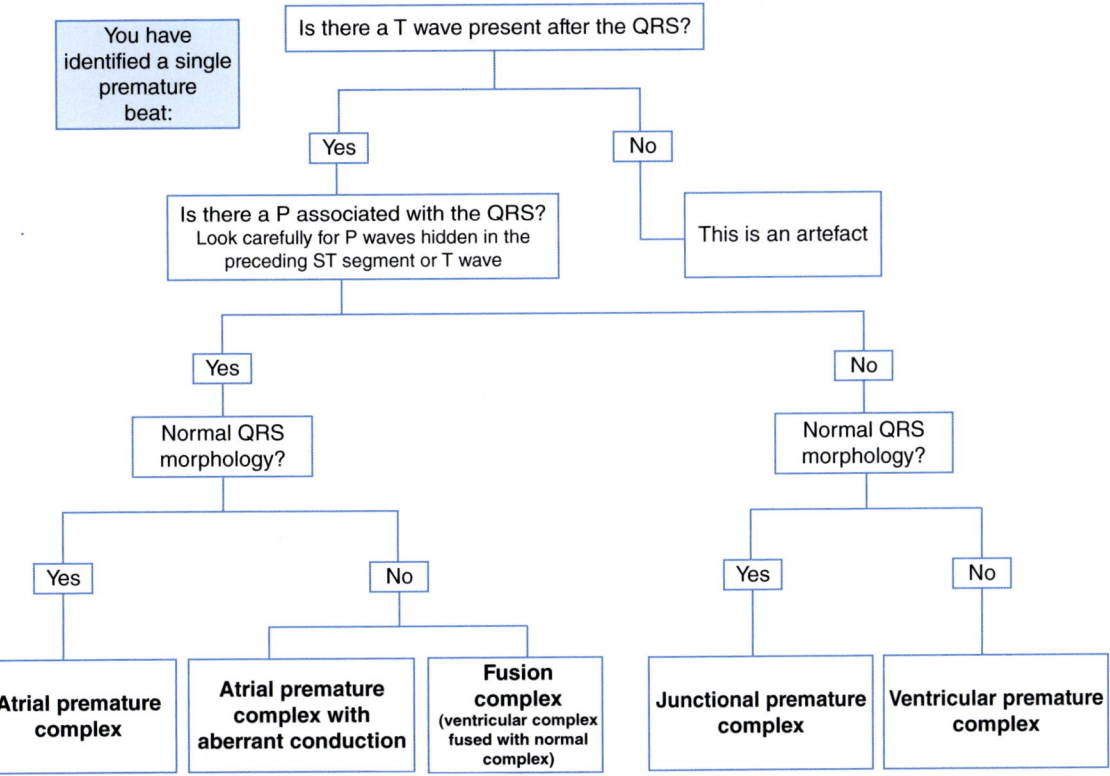

Fig. 4.1. Decision-tree algorithm following identification of a premature beat.

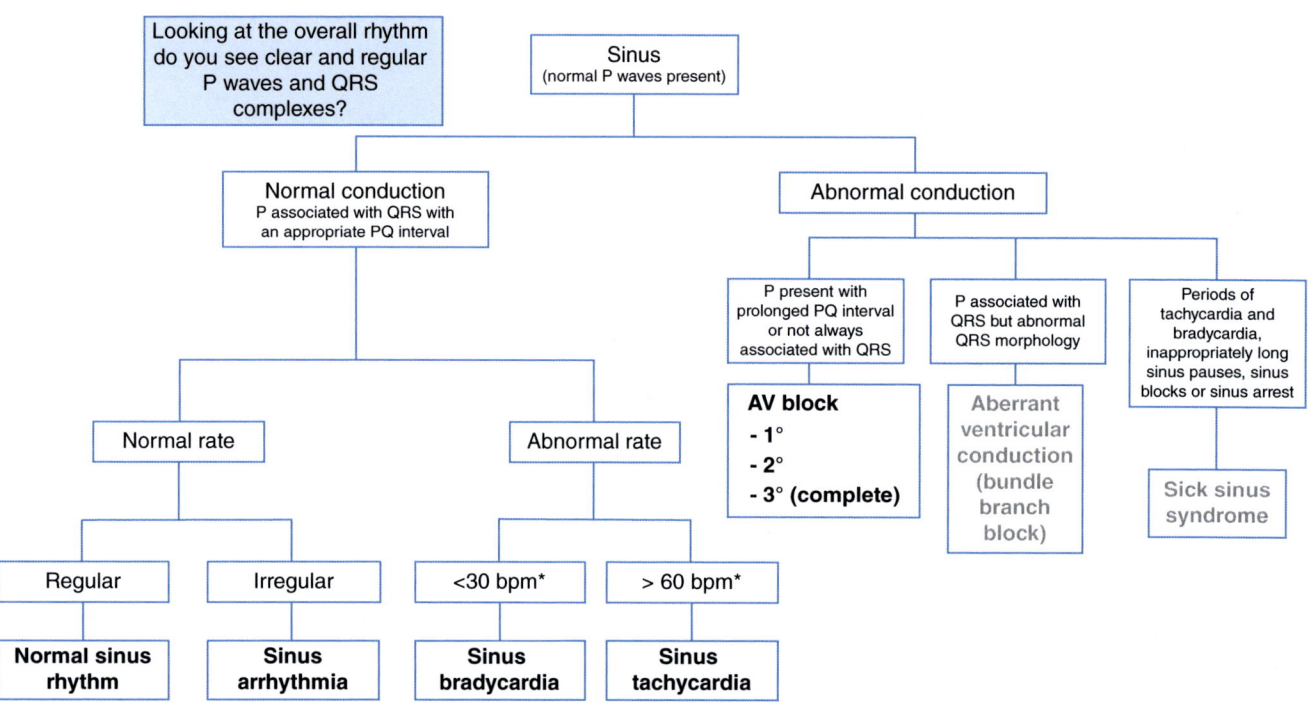

Fig. 4.2. Decision tree algorithm if you suspect the underlying rhythm to be sinus in origin (P waves must be present). The grey text indicates problems uncommonly encountered in equine ECG interpretation.

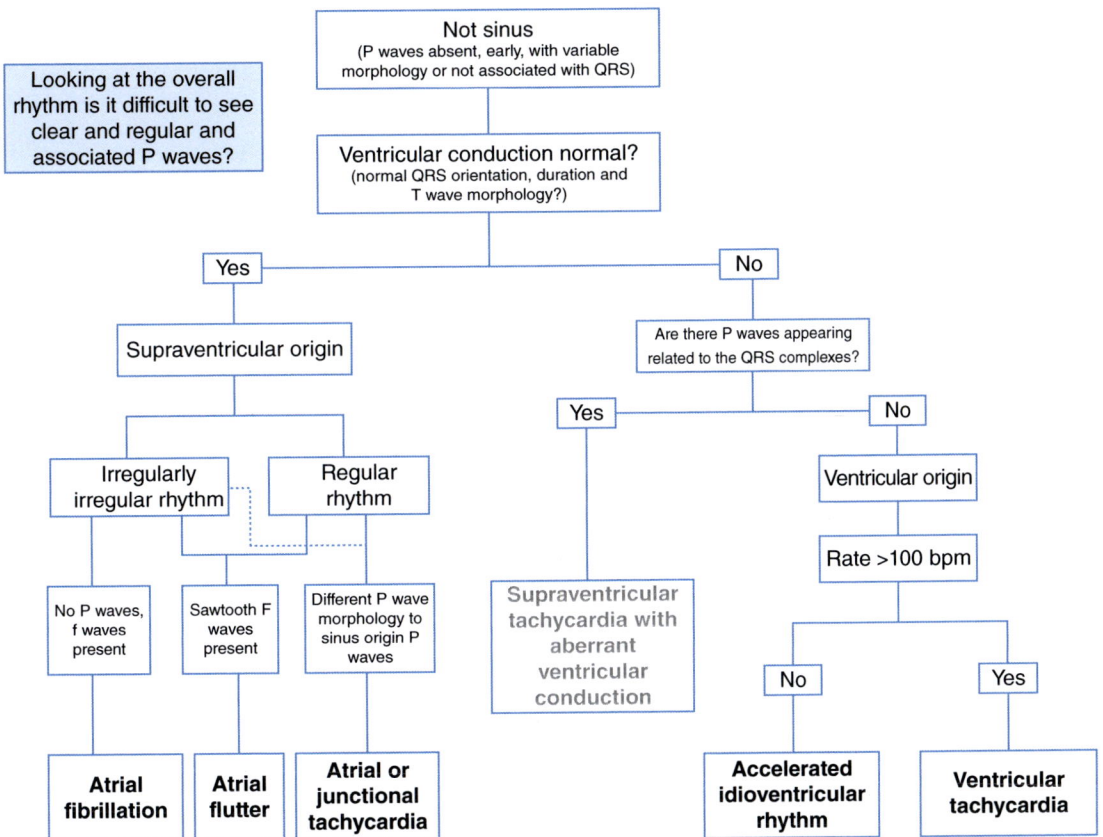

Fig. 4.3. Decision tree algorithm if you suspect the underlying rhythm NOT to be sinus in origin (P waves are absent, irregular, have variable morphology or do not appear to relate to the QRS complexes). The grey text indicates problems uncommonly encountered in equine ECG interpretation. The dotted line indicates a less common presentation.

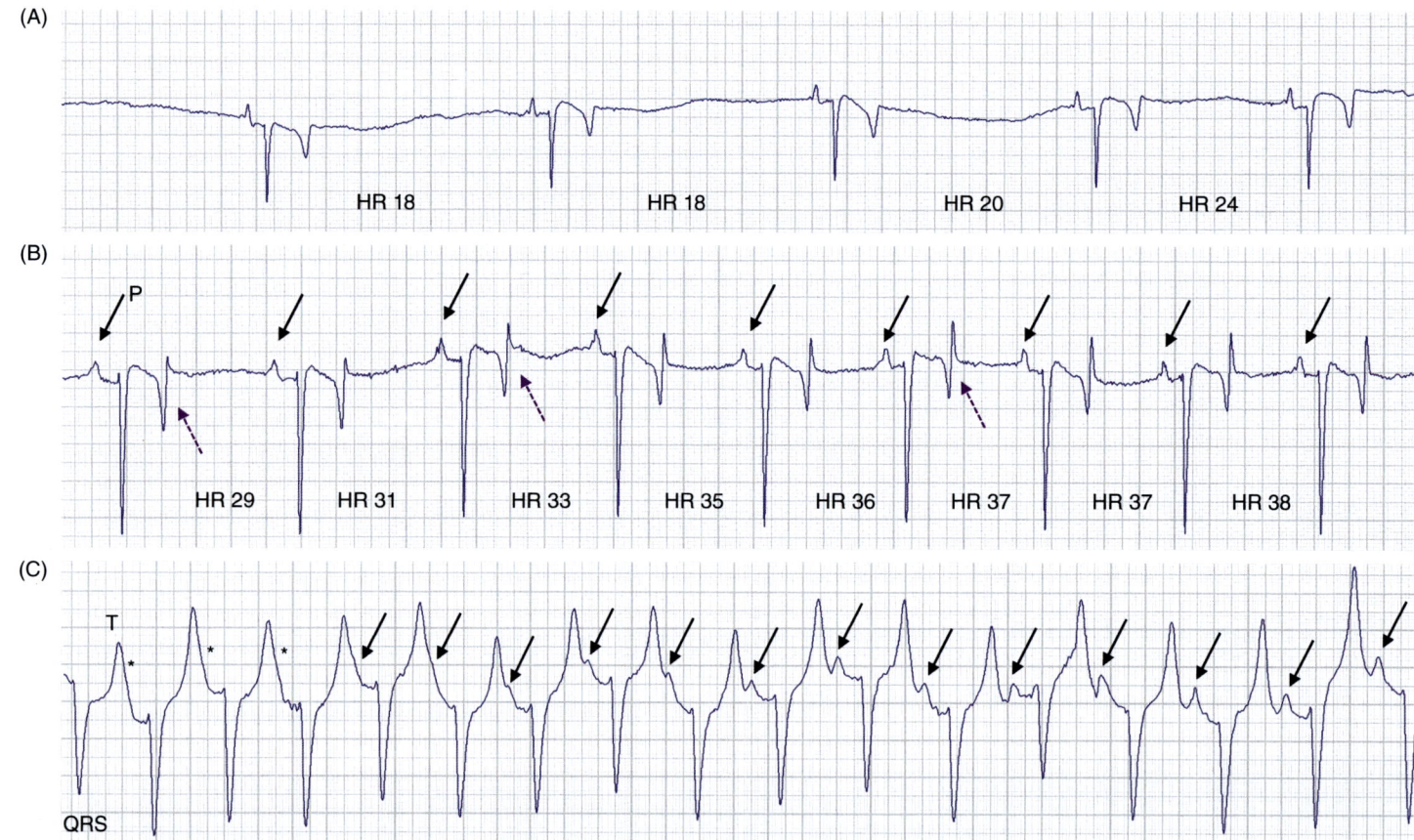

Fig. 4.4. See caption page 45

Sinus pause and sinus block

A sinus pause is an abrupt slowing of the sinus rate, often as a result of tonic vagal inhibition. A sinus block occurs when a sinus impulse is not transmitted out of the SA node, and will result in a PP interval that is twice that of the previous two beats (Fig. 4.5).

AV blocks

Arrhythmias resulting from delayed or absent AV node conduction are a common finding in healthy horses at rest and after exercise.

A first-degree AV block is a prolonged AV node conduction, resulting in a PQ interval duration of more than 400 ms in a 500 kg horse (Schwarzwald *et al.*, 2012). The P:QRS ratio is normal (1:1). An example is seen in Fig. 4.6.

In a second-degree AV block, the normal sinus impulse fails to be conducted through the AV node, with no resulting QRS or ventricular activation. This is seen in Figs 4.5 and 4.6 (see also Fig. 1.3B in Chapter 1). It is common in horses to block one or two complexes in a row; however, blocking three or more QRS complexes is called a 'high-grade or advanced' second-degree AV block and is considered abnormal (Fig. 4.7). Two types of second-degree AV block have been described: (i) Mobitz type 1 (or Wenckebach) where the PR interval gradually increases until conduction across the AV node is blocked and no QRS is recorded; and (ii) Mobitz type 2 where the PR interval is constant before a dropped beat occurs. Both types can be observed in horses, and unlike in human or small-animal medicine, a Mobitz type 2 AV block does not appear to be associated with an increased risk of progression to complete heart block.

All physiological arrhythmias should disappear immediately with stress or exercise, but can return rapidly during the heart-rate deceleration phase.

Fig. 4.4. (A) Sinus bradycardia with sinus arrhythmia. Normal P-QRS-T morphology is seen with a slight increase in heart rate (HR) towards the end of the ECG trace. Paper speed: 25 mm/s. (B) Sinus arrhythmia. There are normal P-QRS-T complexes with a slight increase in HR towards the end of the ECG trace. As the HR increases, small changes in P-wave (black arrows) and T-wave (purple dashed arrows) morphology are observed. Paper speed: 25 mm/s. (C) Sinus tachycardia. There are normal P-QRS-T waves observed; however, at higher HRs, it is difficult to see the P waves buried in the end of the preceding T wave (*). As the HR slows, the P waves become apparent (black arrows). Note the larger positive T waves, a normal finding at higher HRs on an equine surface ECG. Paper speed: 50 mm/s.

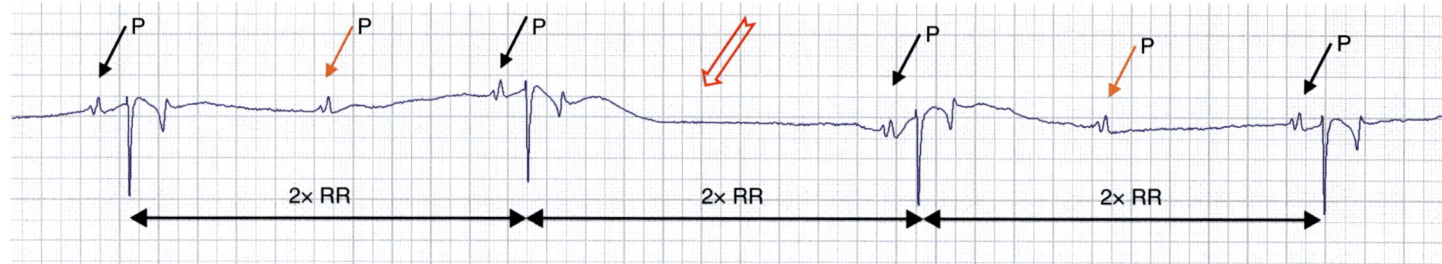

Fig. 4.5. A combination of second-degree atrioventricular blocks (orange arrows) and a sinus block (red arrow) with an underlying sinus arrhythmia (variable PP intervals). The RR intervals are twice as long as normal (2× RR; double-ended arrows). Paper speed: 25 mm/s.

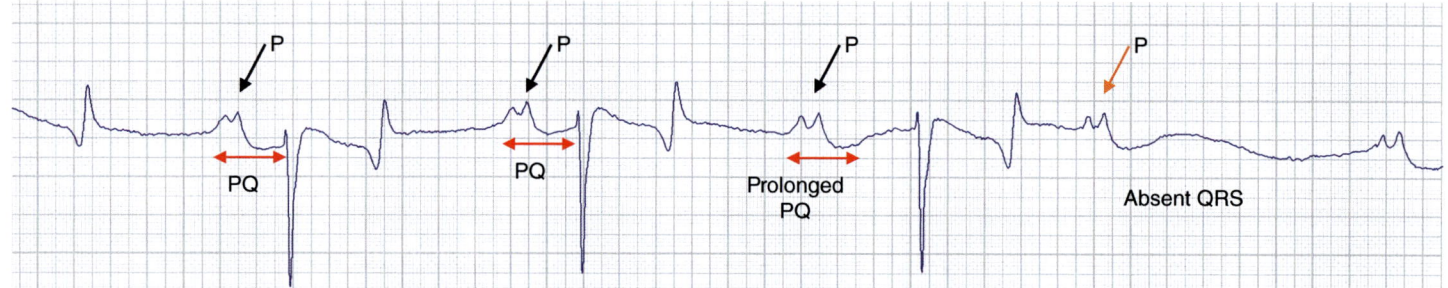

Fig. 4.6. First- and second-degree atrioventricular blocks. Note the present P waves (black arrows), increasing PQ interval (the third PQ interval is greater than 400 ms; red double-ended arrows represent the 'normal' PQ interval of the first complex) and that the fourth P wave (orange arrow) is not followed by a QRS complex. This is an example of the Mobitz type 1 (Wenckebach) pattern. Paper speed: 50 mm/s.

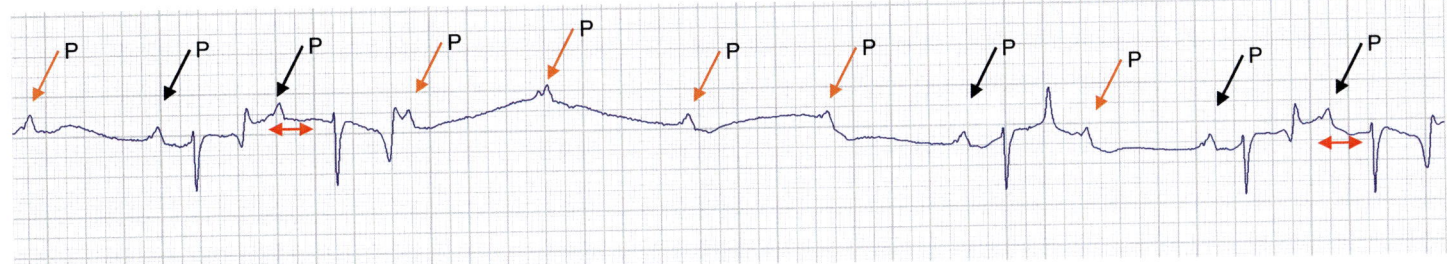

Fig. 4.7. High-grade second-degree atrioventricular (AV) blocks. Here, there are four non-conducted P waves in a row (orange arrows). In addition, there is variable PQ prolongation (red double-ended arrows indicate the shortest or 'normal' PQ interval of the first complex). This ECG was recorded at the walk, where it would be expected that vagally mediated AV blocks would disappear, indicating that this rhythm is probably related to pathological damage within the conduction system. Paper speed: 25 mm/s.

Pathological Arrhythmias

Abnormal sinus rhythm generation or conduction

Sinus arrest
Sinus arrest is a failure of the SA node to generate an impulse, resulting in absent P waves on an ECG. A ventricular escape rhythm will be present until the SA node recovers. This rhythm can be difficult to differentiate from atrial standstill (see below).

Sick sinus syndrome
Although a relatively common diagnosis in small-animal and human cardiology, sick sinus syndrome is rarely reported in horses (van Loon *et al.*, 2002). Sick sinus syndrome refers to a collection of abnormalities of SA node function, including sinus bradycardia,

sinus arrest or sinus block, at times in combination with paroxysms of atrial tachyarrhythmias or slow atrial and ventricular rates (bradycardia–tachycardia syndrome).

Third-degree AV block

Third-degree (complete) heart block is where normal P waves are not conducted through the AV node, and therefore the atrial and ventricular activity becomes completely independent (AV dissociation). The atrial rate is faster than the ventricular rate, while the escape rhythm originates from a junctional or ventricular subsidiary pacemaker, resulting in abnormal QRS morphology, usually at a much slower rate (12–20 bpm) (Luethy *et al.*, 2017). Figure 4.8 provides an example.

Atrial standstill

Atrial standstill is a lack of ECG evidence of atrial depolarization. This results in an absence of P waves on the ECG (Fig. 4.9). The most common presentation of atrial standstill is with hyperkalaemia or digitalis toxicity, where the impulse generated in the SA node is

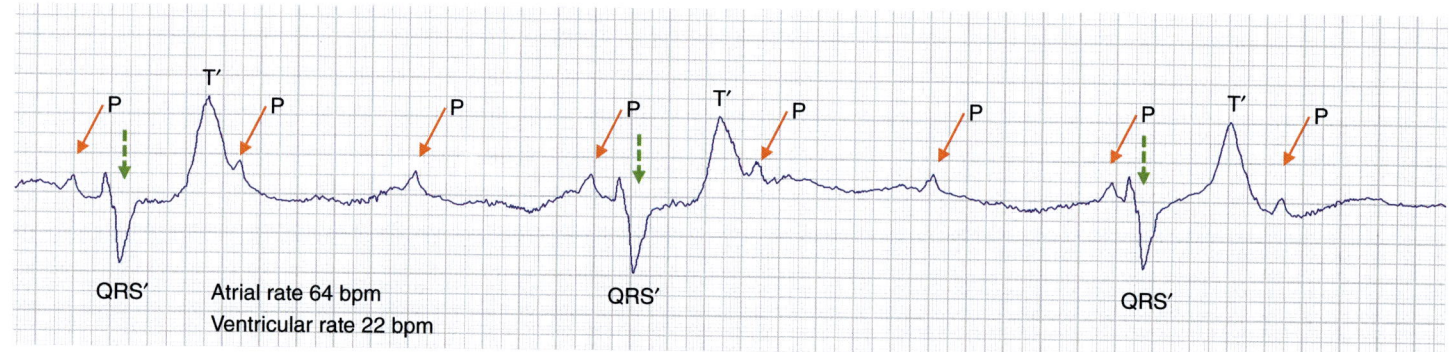

Fig. 4.8. Third-degree (complete) atrioventricular block with a ventricular escape rhythm. There is a mild sinus tachycardia (atrial rate 64 bpm), but all P waves are non-conducted (orange arrows), while wide, abnormal-looking QRS complexes are present at a much lower rate (ventricular rate 22 bpm; green dashed arrows). Paper speed: 50 mm/s.

transmitted to the AV node and ventricle via inter-nodal pathways and Bachman's bundle within the atrial myocardium, but widespread atrial depolarization does not occur. If electrolyte abnormalities are the cause, then other ECG morphology changes can be seen (i.e. wide QRS complex or tall 'tented' T waves).

Bundle branch block

A bundle branch block is a disruption of impulse conduction from between the bundle of His, through either the left or right bundle branches to the Purkinje fibres. This can occur intermittently or permanently, and affects one or both bundle branches. If one bundle is blocked, the ventricles will not depolarize simultaneously, but the ventricle of the blocked bundle will depolarize more slowly due to the impulse being transmitted from cell to cell rather than rapidly via the normal conduction system. With only a three-lead surface ECG, it is not possible to determine the origin of the bundle branch block; a 12-lead ECG is required for this. The typical ECG characteristics include evidence of a supraventricular origin (i.e. not a complex originating in the ventricles) and a wide ± abnormal QRS morphology. An example is seen in Fig. 4.10.

Accessory pathways

Accessory pathways (conduction bridges between the atrial and ventricular tissue other than the AV node) are rarely reported in the horse. An accessory pathway can potentially conduct the electrical impulse more rapidly than the normal, slower, AV nodal tissue, resulting in

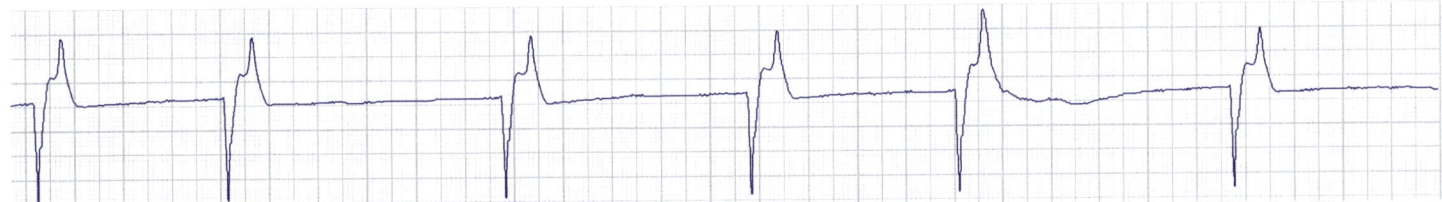

Fig. 4.9. Atrial standstill. No P waves are present. The ventricular rate is 30 bpm with some variation between RR intervals. The QRS complexes appear narrow, but the ST segment and T wave appear abnormal, with a very tall T wave present. Paper speed: 25 mm/s. (ECG courtesy of Professor C. Schwarzwald, University of Zurich, with permission.)

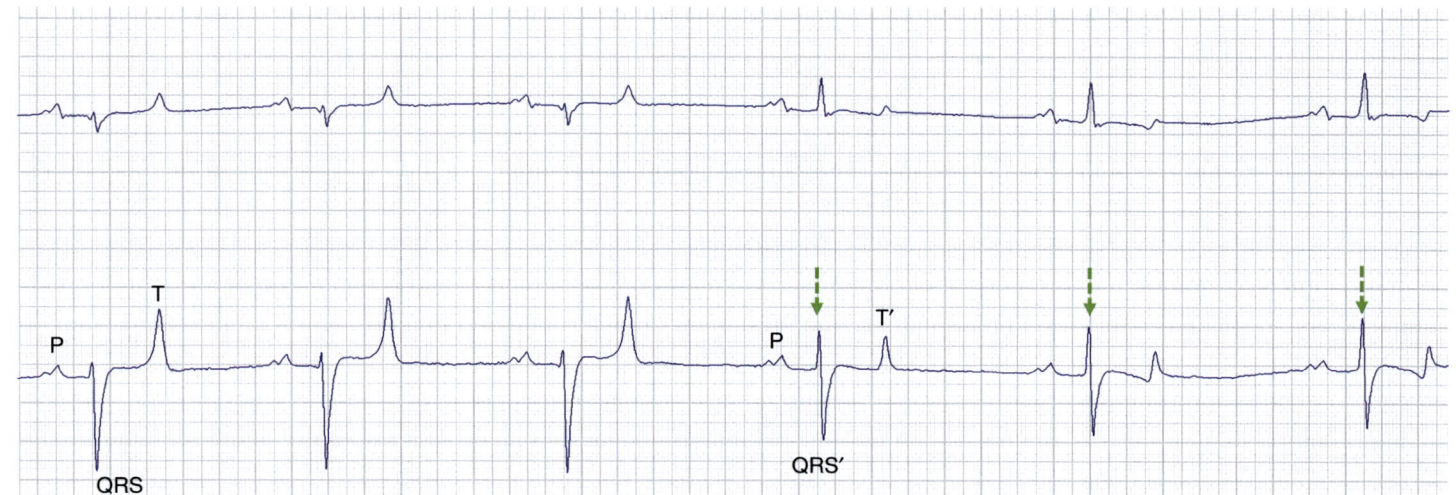

Fig. 4.10. Bundle branch block (BBB). Three normal P-QRS-T complexes are seen on the left. The following three complexes have similar P waves; however, the QRS-T complexes appear different (RS morphology, green dashed arrows). There is a regular and appropriate PR interval with no evidence of atrioventricular dissociation. In this horse, the BBB was occurring intermittently and was heart-rate dependent (normal conduction at higher rates, BBB during heart-rate decelerations or at lower heart rates). Paper speed: 50 mm/s.

ventricular pre-excitation. The classic ECG features are a shortened PR interval, a delta wave (present at the onset of the QRS complex) and different QRS morphology (with a longer duration) compared with normal. This abnormal conduction pathway can create a circus movement between the pathway and the AV node, resulting in a macro re-entry supraventricular arrhythmia. In addition, in cases of atrial fibrillation, conduction of the fibrillation waves to the ventricles can occur via the pathway, resulting in a rapid ventricular response rate (Jesty *et al.*, 2011). In human medicine, both of these scenarios are associated with an increased risk of an adverse event, particularly during exercise. Little is known about the risk of these arrhythmias in horses (Viu *et al.*, 2018).

Supraventricular arrhythmias

Supraventricular rhythms originate from myocardial tissue above the bundle of His, typically within the atria, myocardial sleeves of the vena cava and pulmonary veins, or in the region above the AV node. These rhythms can be classified as: (i) isolated atrial premature complexes (see Fig. 2.3A and Figs 3.3C, D in Chapters 2 and 3); (ii) atrial tachycardia (three or more consecutive atrial premature complexes); (iii) atrial flutter (a single macro re-entry wave over a fixed pathway); or (iv) atrial fibrillation (chaotic, multiple micro re-entry wavelets). It can be difficult to characterize the exact features of atrial tachycardia and atrial flutter on a surface ECG, and therefore, when in doubt, it is better to classify them broadly as atrial tachycardia. These rhythms can be non-sustained (paroxysmal) or sustained (lasting for more than 30 s).

Atrial tachycardia

Arising from ectopic foci in the atrial myocardium, atrial tachycardias in horses can be regular (when conducted 1:1) or irregular (when variable AV conduction occurs). An example of atrial tachycardia is seen in Fig. 4.11. The P waves will have a different morphology from those complexes originating from the SA node (van Steenkiste *et al.*, 2019). Paroxysmal atrial tachycardias typically have an abrupt onset and reversion to sinus rhythm, which is useful when differentiating them from a period of sinus tachycardia (where the rhythm gradually accelerates and decelerates).

Atrial fibrillation

Atrial fibrillation is recognized by replacement of P waves with fibrillation (f) waves, an irregularly irregular RR interval and normal QRS morphology. An example of atrial fibrillation is shown in Fig. 4.12. The requirements for the development of atrial fibrillation are described in Box 4.1.

The atrial fibrillation rate is between 300 and 600 cycles/min; however, with the horse typically having high vagal tone, the AV node blocks most of these impulses, resulting in a fairly normal ventricular rate (but not rhythm) when measured over a longer duration (30–60 s). With conditions of increased sympathetic tone (and withdrawal of parasympathetic tone) such as stress, exercise or with underlying heart disease, the AV nodal conduction of these atrial fibrillation wavelets can increase, resulting in a higher ventricular response rate. An example of this, secondary to heart disease, is seen in Fig. 4.14. These higher ventricular rates can sound more regular during auscultation, but evaluation of the ECG will confirm irregular RR intervals, even during peak exercise.

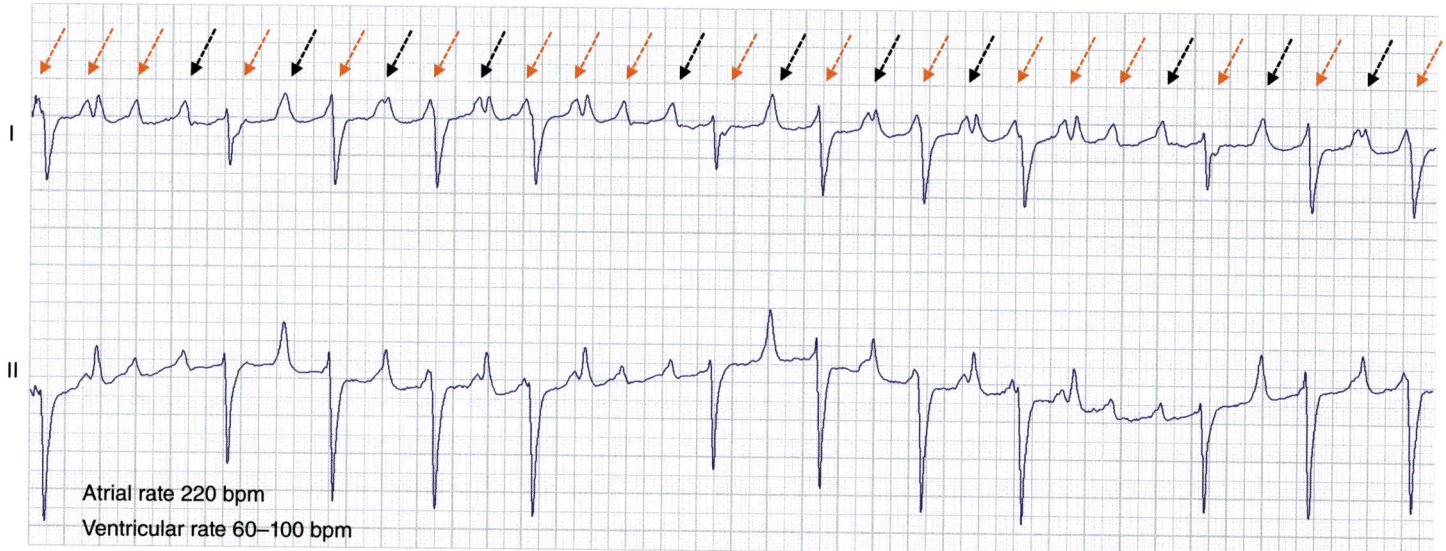

Fig. 4.11. Atrial tachycardia with periods of 2:1 and 4:1 ventricular conduction. Non-sinus-origin P′ waves are observed (atrial rate 220 bpm); those that are conducted to the ventricle are represented by black dashed arrows. Those P′ waves that are not conducted are identified by orange dashed arrows. The ventricular rhythm is regularly irregular (ventricular rate 60–100 bpm). Paper speed: 50 mm/s.

In addition to a rapid ventricular response with increasing sympathetic tone, approximately 30% of horses with atrial fibrillation show evidence of intermittent abnormal QRS morphology and R-on-T phenomenon (Verheyen *et al.*, 2013). An example of this was shown during an exercising ECG in Fig. 2.5A in Chapter 2.

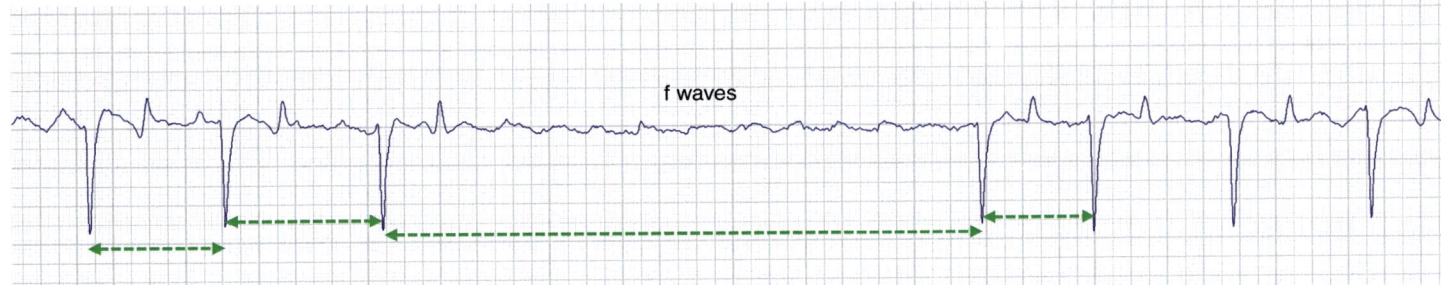

Fig. 4.12. Atrial fibrillation. No P waves can be identified. Instead, fibrillation (f) waves can be seen. The RR interval is highly variable (green dashed double-ended arrows) resulting in an irregularly irregular rhythm. The QRS morphology is normal. The average ventricular rate in this segment is approximately 50 bpm. Paper speed: 50 mm/s.

Box 4.1. Requirements for the development of atrial fibrillation.

- Trigger (e.g. an atrial premature complex, as shown in Fig. 4.13).
- A large enough atrial myocardium ('substrate') to sustain the electrical impulse.
- Favourable electrophysiological conditions (e.g. high vagal tone shortens the atrial refractory period).

Atrial flutter

Atrial flutter is a form of re-entry tachycardia that is initiated and sustained within the atrial myocardium. Similar to atrial fibrillation, the AV node controls the conduction of the impulses to the ventricle. Atrial waveforms can resemble the teeth of a saw and are referred to as flutter (F) waves (e.g. Fig. 14.4B). On an equine surface ECG, it can be very difficult to differentiate atrial flutter from atrial fibrillation or atrial tachycardia. Electro-anatomical mapping of the equine myocardium is currently the only way to differentiate clearly the origin of these arrhythmias.

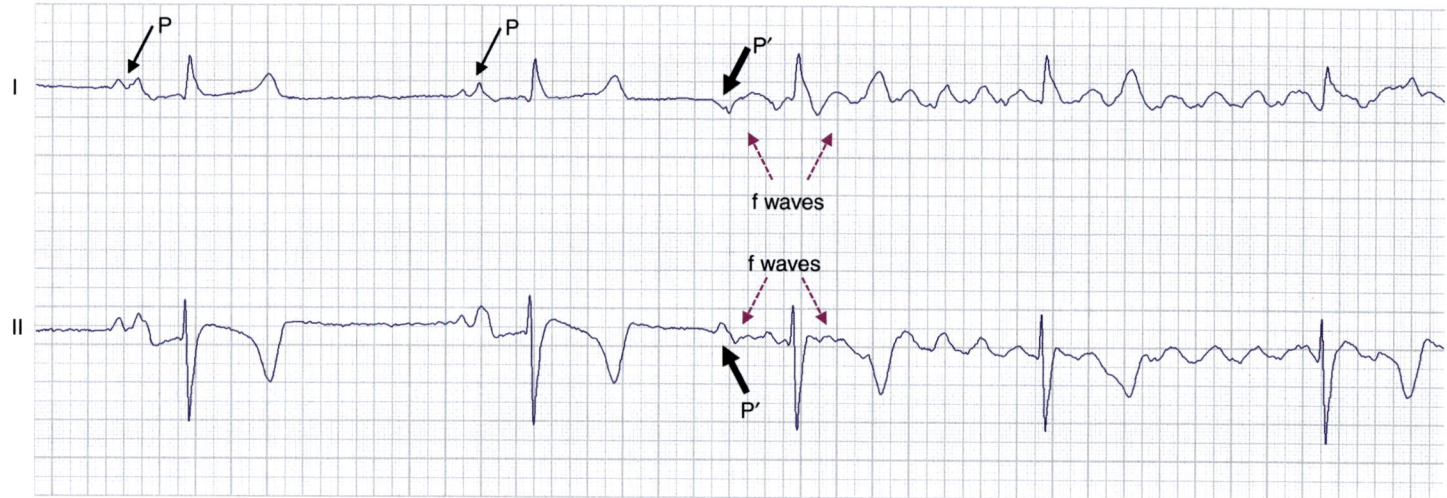

Fig. 4.13. The onset of atrial fibrillation. An atrial premature complex (bold arrow) is seen triggering atrial fibrillation. Fibrillation waves (purple dashed arrows) are seen occurring immediately after the premature P′ wave. The ventricular rhythm immediately becomes irregularly irregular. Paper speed: 50 mm/s.

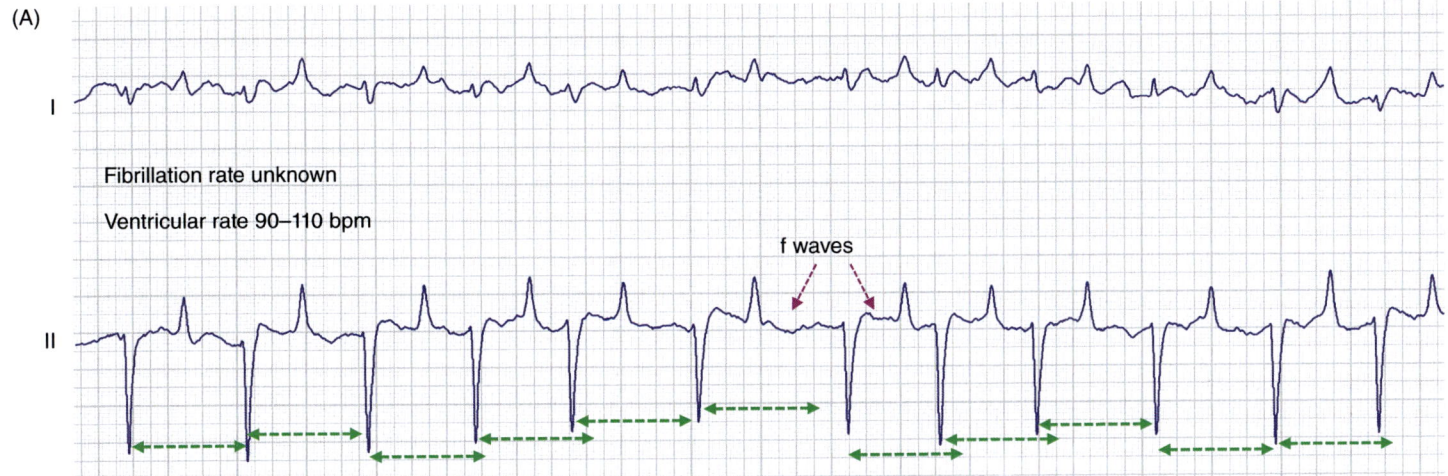

Fig. 4.14. (A) Atrial fibrillation with a rapid ventricular conduction rate. Here, the ventricular rate is 90–110 bpm. This is caused by decreasing vagal tone and increasing sympathetic tone, as seen with stress, exercise or serious heart disease. In this case, severe myocarditis was present. On the ECG, no P waves are identified. It can be difficult to see fibrillation (f) waves (purple dashed arrows) at higher heart rates, but the RR intervals remain irregularly irregular (green dashed double-ended arrows equal to the length of the first RR interval). Paper speed: 50 mm/s.

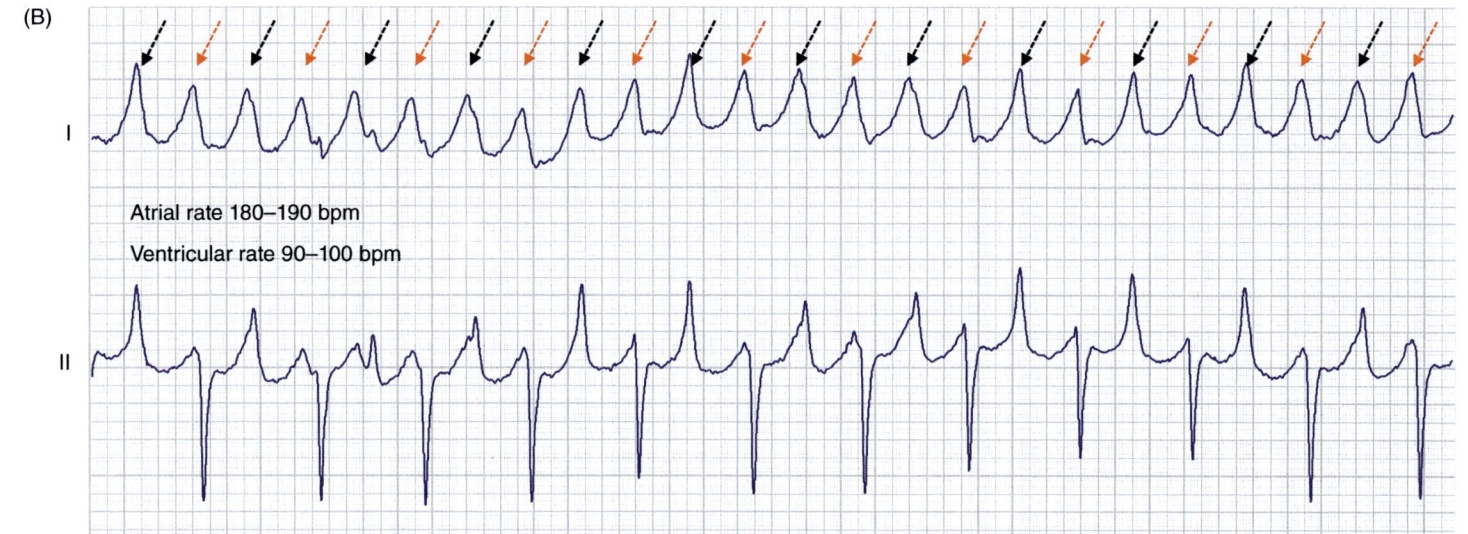

Fig. 4.14. Continued.
(B) The same horse as seen in Fig. 4.14A, 3 h later. The atrial activity can be seen spontaneously organizing into an atrial 'flutter'-like appearance (dashed arrows). There is 2:1 conduction, where every second 'flutter' (F) wave is conducted to the ventricle, resulting in a normal QRS complex (black dashed arrows), while the other F waves (orange dashed arrows) are not conducted. The atrial 'flutter' rate is 180–190 bpm, while the ventricular rate is 90–100 bpm. Often during cardioversion of atrial fibrillation with quinidine sulfate, similar ECG changes are observed leading up to conversion to sinus rhythm. Paper speed: 50 mm/s.

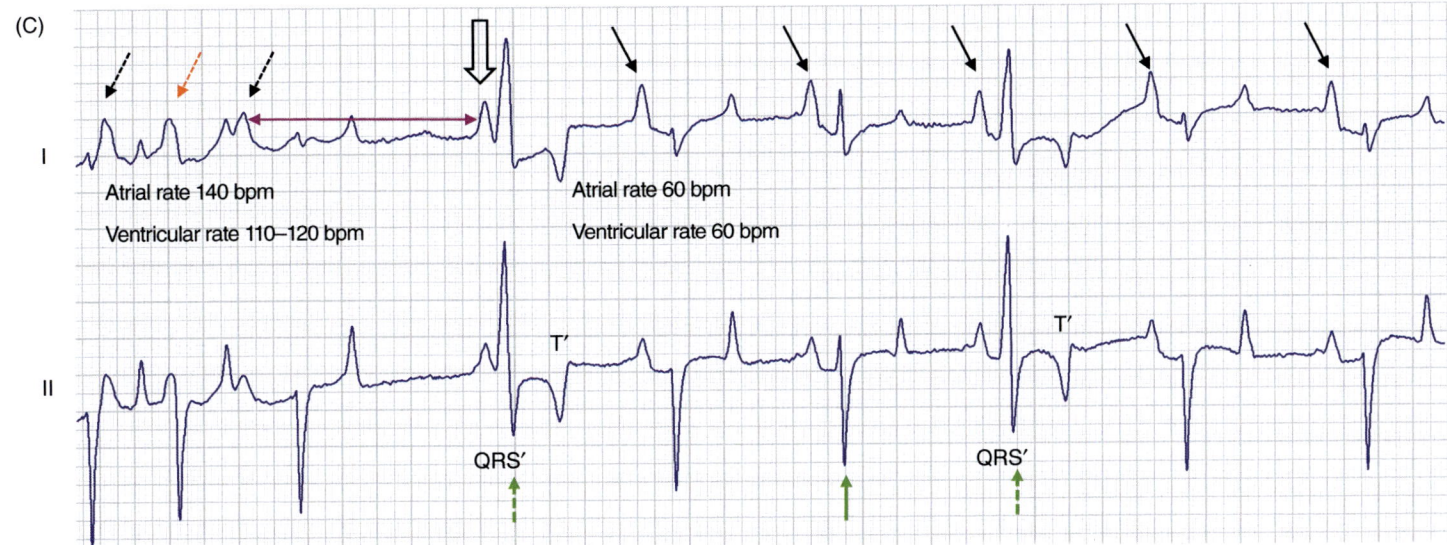

(C)

I

Atrial rate 140 bpm

Ventricular rate 110–120 bpm

Atrial rate 60 bpm

Ventricular rate 60 bpm

II

T′

T′

QRS′

QRS′

Fig. 4.14. Continued.
(C) The same horse as seen in Figs 4.14A and 4.14B, 1 min after Fig. 4.14B was recorded. Spontaneous conversion to sinus rhythm is observed. There is slowing of the atrial 'flutter' rate to 140 bpm (black and orange dashed arrows), before a period of no atrial activity (purple double-ended arrow). The sinoatrial node activity then starts (black open arrow) and regular P waves can be identified following this (black arrows). There are also two ventricular complexes present (green dashed arrows) and one probable fusion or aberrantly conducted complex (green arrow), while the remaining QRS complexes appear normal. Paper speed: 50 mm/s.

Accelerated idiojunctional rhythm and junctional tachycardia

Junctional rhythms occur when the AV nodal tissue takes over the rhythm from the SA node. These rhythms are uncommonly observed in equine ECGs. Atrial depolarization can occur from retrograde conduction of the impulse backwards to the atrial myocardium, and therefore P waves can be immediately before, during (hidden in the QRS) or after the QRS complex. As the impulse will travel via the normal pathways to the ventricular myocardium, the QRS morphology will be the same as for a sinus rhythm. When the junctional rate is between 60 and 100 bpm, these are described as accelerated idiojunctional rhythms, while rates over 100 bpm are described as junctional tachycardias. An example of an idiojunctional rhythm is seen in Fig. 4.15.

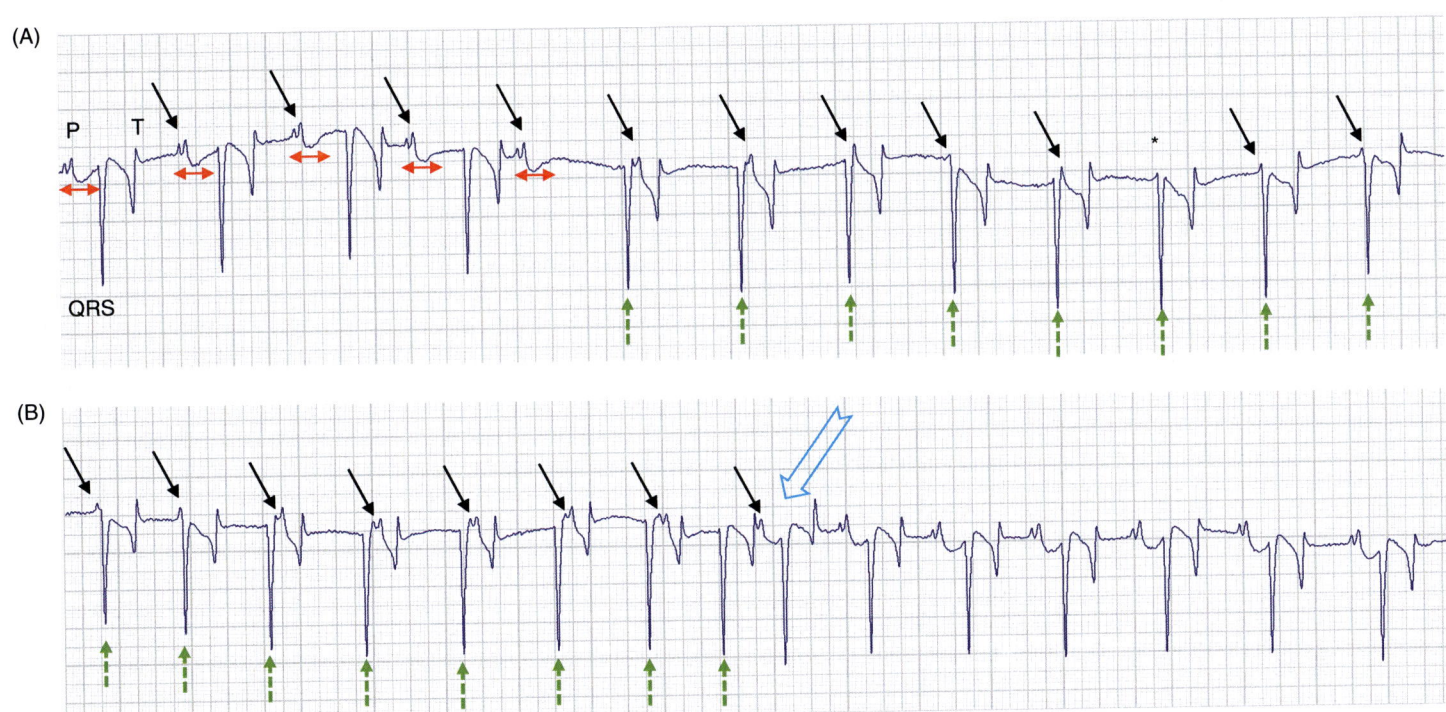

Fig. 4.15. Onset (A) and cessation (B) of an accelerated idiojunctional rhythm. A sinus rhythm with progressive lengthening of the PR interval (first-degree AV block; red double-ended arrows) is seen initially. A second-degree AV block then occurs and the accelerated idiojunctional rhythm takes over. Regular P waves can be seen in the QRS complex or ST segment of the junctional complexes (black arrows), although it can be difficult to identify all the P waves clearly (*). The junctional QRS complexes (green dashed arrows) are identical to those originating from the sinus rhythm as they follow the same conduction pathway. The junctional rhythm is terminated when a faster junctional complex occurs in combination with a slowing of the sinus rate, allowing the next P wave to be conducted normally (blue arrow). During this episode, the junctional rhythm persisted for 3 min and reoccurred intermittently over the 24 h period of ECG recording. Paper speed: 25 mm/s.

Ventricular arrhythmias

Ventricular rhythms originate from spontaneous depolarizations of the ventricular myocardium. A ventricular complex can be premature (see Figs 2.3B, 2.5B, 3.2, 3.3A in Chapters 2 and 3) or delayed (ventricular escape, see Fig. 4.8). Ventricular rhythms are characterized by an abnormal QRS size (duration) and/or orientation when compared with the QRS complex originating from a sinus impulse. Because the ventricular depolarization was abnormal, the repolarization will also be different, resulting in T-wave morphology alterations. A ventricular complex will lack a preceding, associated P wave with a consistent and appropriate PQ interval. Those impulses originating from high in the bundle of His will have a similar QRS morphology to the normal sinus complexes and will be difficult to differentiate from junctional complexes.

Accelerated idioventricular rhythm and ventricular tachycardia

When more than three consecutive ventricular premature complexes are observed at rates over 100 bpm, this is called ventricular tachycardia (VT). For rates between 60 and 100 bpm, this is known as 'slow VT' or an accelerated idioventricular rhythm (Fig. 4.16). Similar to the supraventricular rhythms, those lasting less than 30 s are described as non-sustained or paroxysmal, while those present for longer periods are considered sustained.

Monomorphic (uniform) VT has a single QRS-T morphology, while the QRS-T morphology varies in polymorphic (multi-form) VT. Examples are seen in Figs 4.17 and 4.18. When the coupling interval between QRS complexes is short, the subsequent QRS complex occurs before the preceding T wave is complete, resulting in the so-called R-on-T phenomenon. Torsade de pointes describes a specific

Fig. 4.16.

The onset and termination of a period of accelerated idioventricular rhythm that lasted approximately 3 min. An abrupt onset and termination of abnormal rhythm can be seen (blue arrows). The abnormal QRS complexes have a normal polarity in lead II but are much larger and wider than the normal complexes. A different QRS polarity (RS) can be seen in lead III during the period of abnormal rhythm (green dashed arrows). There are P waves wandering in and out of the abnormal QRS complexes (black arrows), indicating atrioventricular dissociation, with an atrial rate starting at 36 bpm and increasing to 48 bpm during the period of abnormal rhythm. The ventricular rate is between 70 and 95 bpm during the period of abnormal ventricular rhythm. Paper speed: 25 mm/s.

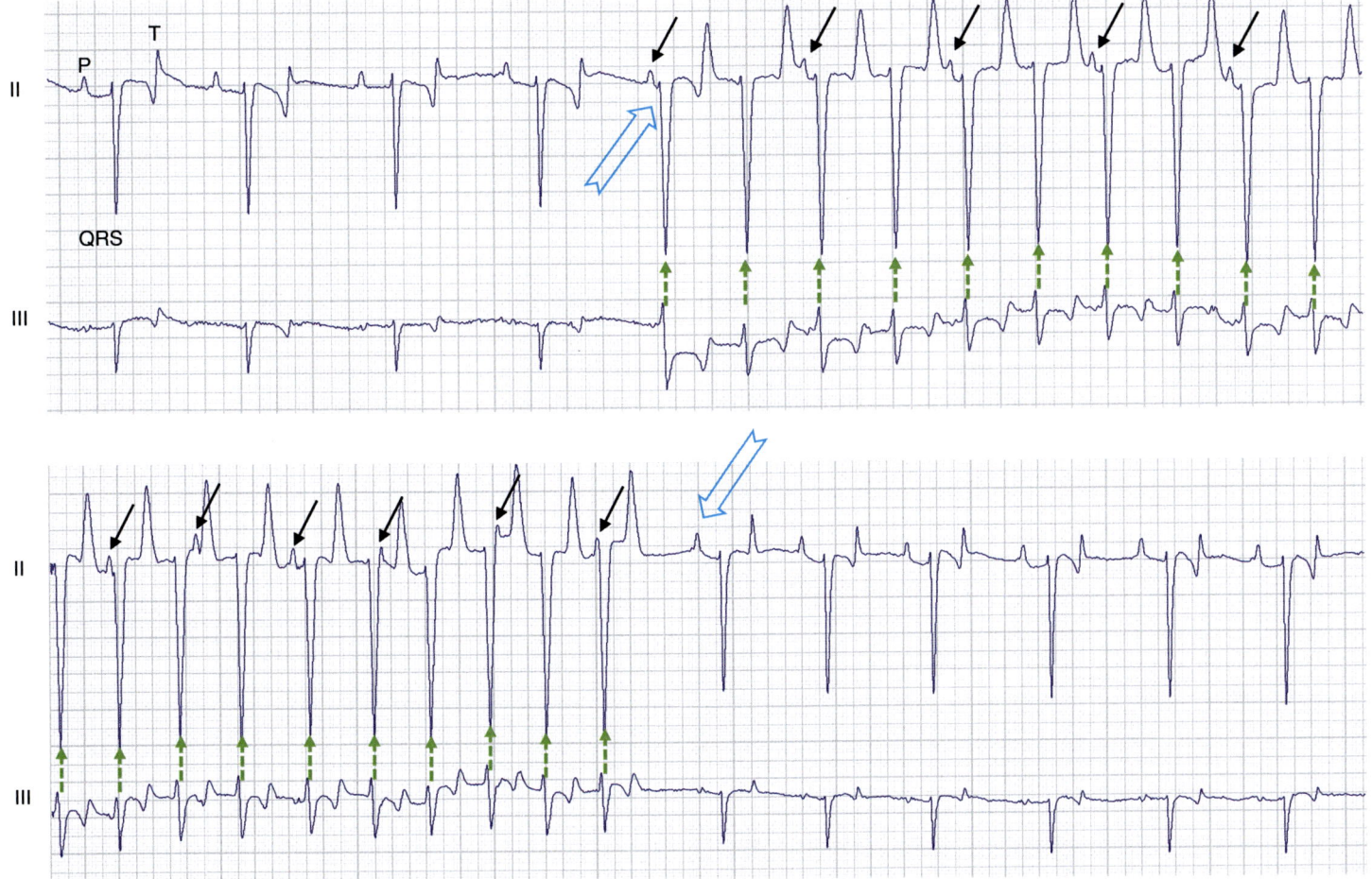

Fig. 4.16.

form of polymorphic VT associated with marked QT prolongation and sinusoidal twisting of the QRS around the isoelectric baseline forming prominent U waves that show beat-to-beat lability. The R-on-T phenomenon and torsade de pointes can both be self-limiting but have the potential to cause electrical instability and to rapidly deteriorate to ventricular fibrillation, which invariably results in cardiac arrest in the horse.

Ventricular fibrillation

Ventricular fibrillation is a chaotic rhythm with no organized myocardial contraction. There are no P, QRS or T waves distinguishable. It is an invariably fatal rhythm in the horse, even when internal electrical defibrillation is available.

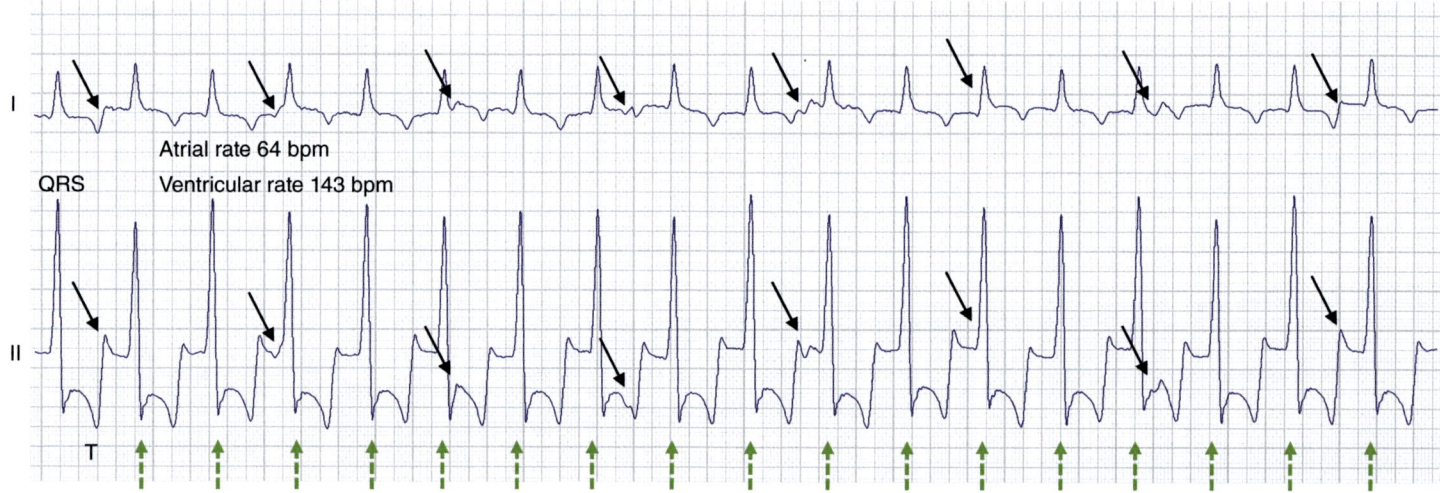

Fig. 4.17. Monomorphic (uniform) ventricular tachycardia with a regular ventricular rate of 143 bpm. Abnormal QRS morphology (Rs) is seen (green dashed arrows) and no normal QRS complexes can be identified. P waves can be found wandering in and out of the QRS complexes (black arrows), indicating atrioventricular dissociation, with an atrial rate slower than the ventricular rate (64 bpm). Paper speed: 50 mm/s.

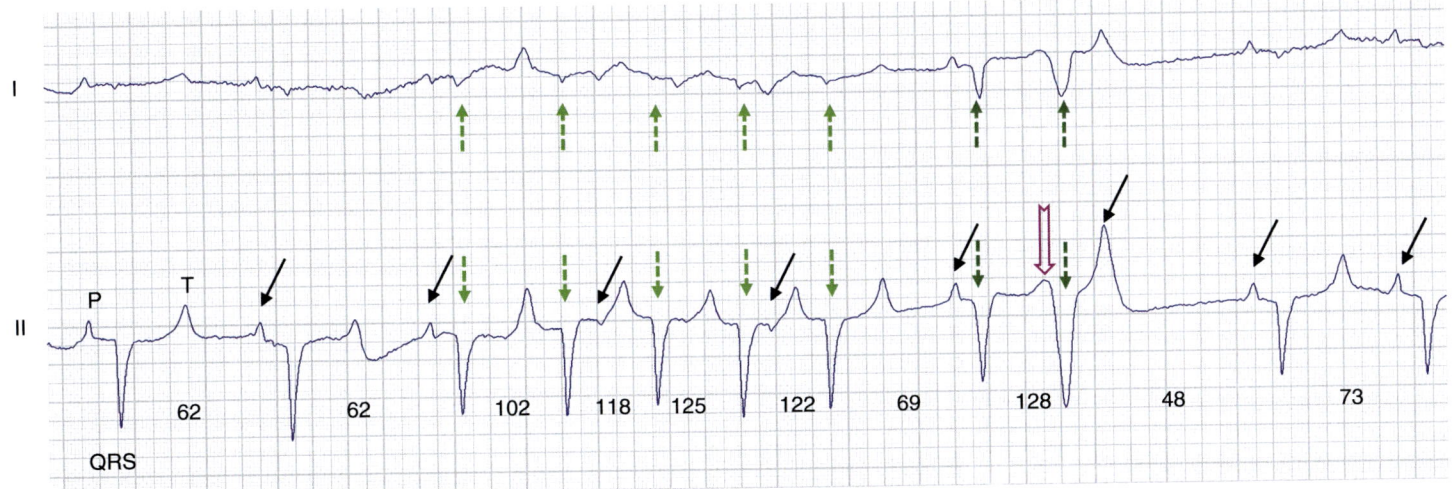

Fig. 4.18. Polymorphic (multi-form) accelerated idioventricular rhythm/ventricular tachycardia. The instantaneous heart rate is displayed below the trace and varies from 62 to 128 bpm. The first five abnormal QRS complexes (light green dashed arrows) are similar in morphology to the normal complexes and could be junctional or high ventricular in origin. The last two abnormal QRS complexes have different morphology (dark green dashed arrows). The last ventricular complex shows R-on-T phenomenon, with the subsequent QRS occurring on the preceding complex's T wave (purple arrow). P waves can be seen wandering through the abnormal QRS complexes (black arrows), indicating atrioventricular dissociation, with an atrial rate of 64 bpm. Paper speed: 50 mm/s.

Therapy

Therapeutic options for equine arrhythmias are limited compared with those available in human or small-animal medicine. This is due to a number of factors, including higher body weight (and therefore costs of medication), poor or variable bioavailability of many oral medications, adverse effects (many of which can be fatal) and a lack of evidence-based treatment recommendations for those arrhythmias occurring infrequently. It is important to remember that all anti-arrhythmic medications can also be pro-arrhythmic, potentially worsening the arrhythmias already present.

Figure 5.1 indicates the four classes of anti-arrhythmic agents, as classified by the original Vaughan Williams system, and their effects on the action potential of both ventricular and nodal tissue. The four classes are sodium (Na^+) channel blockers (class 1), β-blockers (class II), potassium (K^+) channel blockers (class III) and calcium (Ca^{2+}) channel blockers (class IV). Examples and indications for the commonly used equine anti-arrhythmic drugs are presented in Tables 5.1–5.4.

The indications for immediate treatment of arrhythmias are presented in Box 5.1.

Atrial fibrillation is the most commonly identified pathological arrhythmia in horses; specific details regarding treatment are presented in Box 5.2 and in Fig. 5.2 (Reef *et al.*, 1995, McGurrin *et al.*, 2008, Decloedt *et al.*, 2015). If therapy with quinidine sulfate is chosen, it is extremely important to monitor the patient closely during and after therapy. Continuous ECG recording (with an ambulatory, telemetric device) should be performed in *every* case. Regular visual assessment of the ECG is essential to monitor for the moment of cardioversion as well as any complications that may occur as a result of therapy (e.g. tachycardia, widening of the QRS complex, R-on-T phenomenon or ventricular arrhythmias). It is not uncommon for a rapid atrial flutter (F)-type rhythm with 2:1 conduction to develop (similar to that seen in Fig. 4.14B in Chapter 4) and this should not be confused with conversion to sinus rhythm. The ECG should be examined closely for any F waves hidden within the QRS complex, ST segment or T wave.

If transvenous electrical cardioversion is chosen as a therapy, the horse should be referred to an appropriate specialist institution offering this as a therapy.

Therapy for bradyarrhythmias depends on identifying the underlying cause and determining whether treatment is indicated. In horses and donkeys with no evidence of underlying structural disease, pacemaker implantation may be necessary to improve cardiac output (Reef *et al.*, 1986; Pibarot *et al.*, 1993; van Loon *et al.*, 2002). Pharmacological therapy for confirmation and temporary treatment of bradyarrhythmias is covered in Table 5.4.

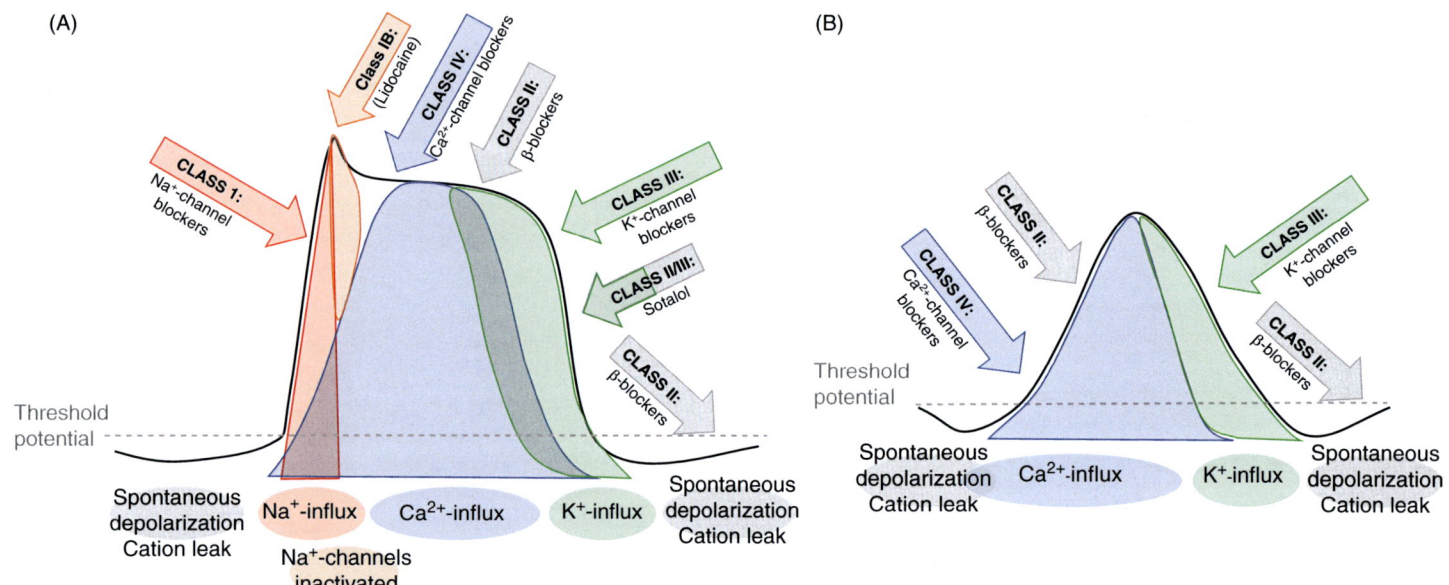

Fig. 5.1. (A) A ventricular action potential. (B) An action potential from nodal tissue. The actions of different classes of anti-arrhythmic drugs are demonstrated in (A) and (B). Class I anti-arrhythmic agents decrease phase 0 of the ventricular action potential caused by the rapid sodium (Na⁺) channels and influx of sodium. The class 1B agent lidocaine binds with the highest affinity to the Na⁺ channels once they are inactivated and does not cause any prolongation of the QRS duration, unlike some of the other class I agents. Class II drugs (β-blockers) have complex actions, including inhibition of spontaneous (phase 4) depolarization and indirect closure of calcium (Ca²⁺) channels. Class III agents block the outward potassium (K⁺) channels, prolonging the action potential and increasing refractoriness. These mediations will result in prolongation of the QT interval. Class IV drugs inhibit the inward Ca²⁺ channels, which are most prominent in nodal tissue, particularly the atrioventricular node. Many of the anti-arrhythmic agents have multiple actions but are classified based on the ion channel that is most affected.

Box 5.1. Indications for treatment of arrhythmias.

- Evidence of haemodynamic compromise:
  - Poor peripheral perfusion (cold extremities, weak pulses)
  - Delayed jugular filling, jugular pulsation or jugular distension
  - Prolonged capillary refill time
  - Reduced urine output
  - Dull mentation
  - Weakness
  - Collapse/syncope
  - Low systemic blood pressure
  - Laboratory evidence of reduced perfusion (e.g. hyperlactataemia or azotaemia).
- Ventricular rate is consistently high (>100 bpm) or extremely low (<20 bpm).
- Polymorphic ventricular complexes are identified.
- R-on-T phenomenon is observed.
- Torsade de pointes.

Box 5.2. Indications for treatment of atrial fibrillation.

- Atrial fibrillation without evidence of relevant, underlying structural heart disease.
- Exercise intolerance or poor performance that can be attributed to atrial fibrillation.
- Excessively high ventricular response rates during stress or exercise (ventricular rates >220 bpm).
- Aberrant QRS conduction or ventricular arrhythmias with the R-on-T phenomenon at higher heart rates.

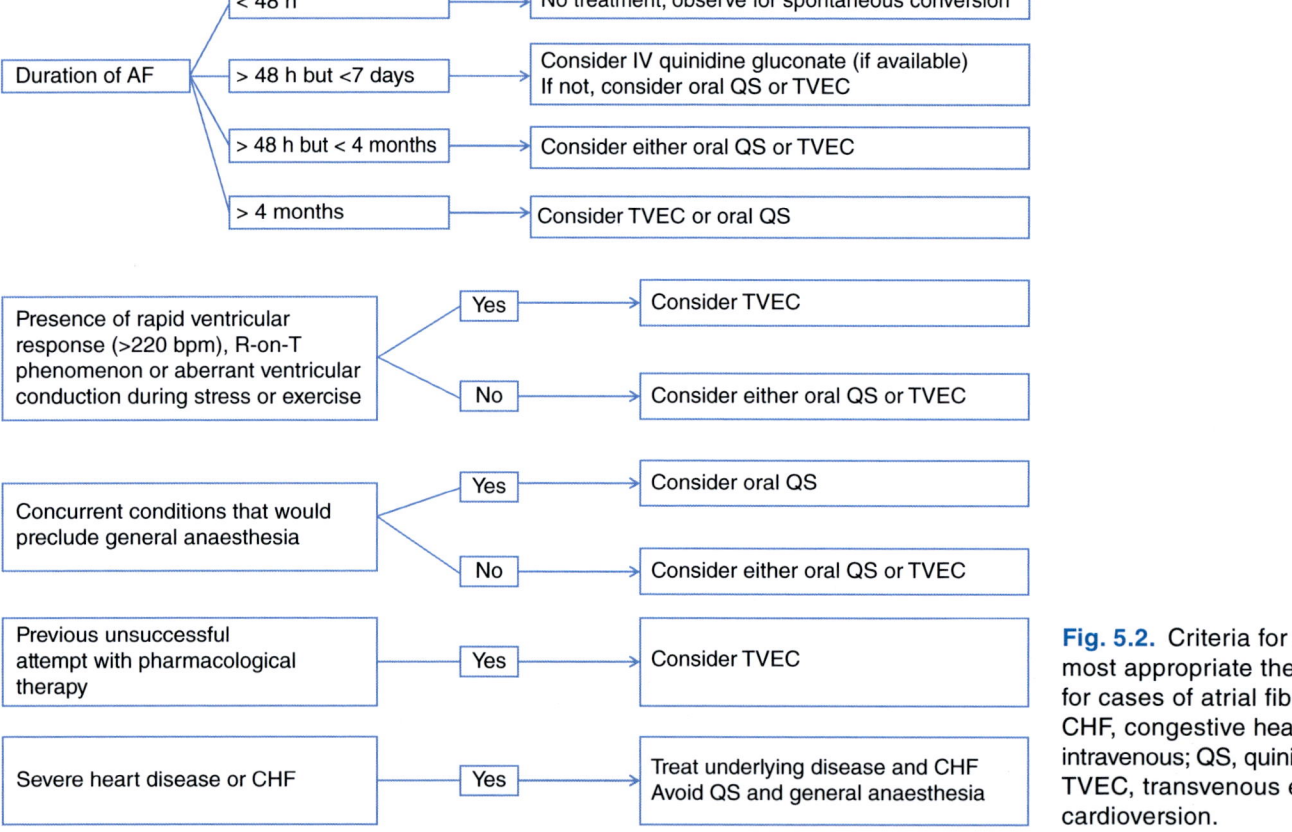

Fig. 5.2. Criteria for deciding the most appropriate therapeutic option for cases of atrial fibrillation (AF). CHF, congestive heart failure; IV, intravenous; QS, quinidine sulfate; TVEC, transvenous electrical cardioversion.

Table 5.1. Anti-arrhythmic drugs for use with sustained supraventricular arrhythmias.

Drug	Drug class	Dose recommendations	Dose for 500 kg bwt	Comments
First-line medication for *rhythm* control for (i) atrial fibrillation and (ii) supraventricular tachycardia (confirmed)				
Quinidine sulfate	Class I$_A$ Na$^+$-channel blocker	22 mg/kg bwt PO by NGT every 2 h for four (max. up to six) doses until converted, adverse or toxic effects, or plasma quinidine concentration >4 μg/mL. Do not exceed 6 doses PO within the first 12 h. Continue if not converted every 6–8 h until converted, adverse or toxic effects, or total dose of 180 mg/kg. **Stop therapy if:** QRS duration exceeds >25% of its pre-treatment value, plasma quinidine concentration >4 μg/ml, or significant adverse reaction or signs of toxicity are observed	11 g per dose	**Use with caution.** *Adverse effects*: commonly, depression, diarrhoea, colic, ataxia, nasal mucosal swelling; less commonly, paraphimosis, urticaria, laminitis. Monitor for: Acceleration of AV conduction, tachycardia, QRS and QT prolongation, VT, torsade de pointes, hypotension, negative inotropism, exacerbation of heart failure, cardiovascular collapse, or sudden death. *Therapeutic drug monitoring*: therapeutic range 2–5 μg/ml (6.2–15.4 μmol/l) 1–2 h after PO administration. *Contraindications*: ventricular tachyarrhythmias, torsade de pointes, untreated heart failure, pre-existing QRS or QT interval prolongation, complete AV block or digitalis intoxication. Use with caution in patients with hypokalaemia, hypomagnesaemia, hypoxia or acid-base disorders. **If therapy with quinidine sulfate is chosen, an IV catheter should be placed, and the emergency drugs required to treat any adverse effects should be available immediately adjacent to the stall, with the appropriate drug doses calculated for the patient's weight**. Transvenous electrical cardioversion could be considered in cases where quinidine sulfate therapy is contraindicated and there is no underlying relevant structural heart disease or heart failure.

Continued

Table 5.1. Continued.

Drug	Drug class	Dose recommendations	Dose for 500 kg bwt	Comments
Second-line medication for *rhythm* control of (i) atrial fibrillation or (ii) supraventricular tachycardia (confirmed)				
Quinidine gluconate	Class I_A Na$^+$-channel blocker	1–2.2 mg/kg bwt IV every 10 min or 0.1–0.22 mg/kg bwt/min CRI up to 12 mg/kg bwt total dose	500 mg–1.1 g every 10 min or 50–110 mg/min CRI; total dose 6 g	**Use with caution.** See adverse reactions and contraindications for quinidine sulfate provided above in the table. For use in acute cases only (<7 days duration). Not available in all regions of the world.
Amiodarone	Class III K$^+$-channel blocker	5 mg/kg bwt/h IV for 1 h, followed by 0.83 mg/kg bwt/h for 23 h; subsequently, 1.9 mg/kg bwt/h for 30 h or to effect	2.5 g for first hour, then 415 mg/h for the next 23 h, then 950 mg/h for additional 30 h	Also class I, II and IV effects. *Adverse reactions*: hind limb weakness, weight shifting, torsade de pointes, SA and AV nodal inhibition, bradycardia, hypotension. Prolonged treatment may affect lungs, liver, heart, thyroid gland, GI tract, eyes, skin and nerves. *Contraindications*: SA node dysfunction, bradycardia, AV block, cardiogenic shock.
Procainamide	Class I_A Na$^+$-channel blocker	1 mg/kg bwt/min IV, up to 20 mg/kg bwt total dose	500 mg/min; total dose 10 g	For use in acute cases only (<7 days duration). *Adverse events*: hypotension, QRS and QT prolongation, negative inotropism, arrhythmia, GI and neurological disorders (similar to but generally less severe than quinidine). *Contraindications*: untreated heart failure, prolonged QRS or QT interval, complete AV block, digitalis intoxication. Use with caution in patients with hypokalaemia, hypomagnesaemia or acid-base disorders.
Propafenone	Class I_C Na$^+$-channel blocker	0.5–1.0 mg/kg bwt in 5% dextrose slowly IV over 5–10 min	250–500 mg IV over 5–10 min	Not commonly available. *Adverse effects*: GI and neurological disorders, bronchospasm, negative inotropism, exacerbation of heart failure, AV block, QRS and QT prolongation, arrhythmias. *Contraindications*: structural heart disease, heart failure, SA or AV node dysfunction.

Continued

Table 5.1. Continued.

Drug	Drug class	Dose recommendations	Dose for 500 kg bwt	Comments
First-line medication for short-duration *rate* control				
Xylazine	α_2-agonist	0.25–0.5 mg/kg bwt slow IV, repeat once if required	125–250 mg IV over 2–3 min	*Adverse effects*: muscle tremors, bradycardia with AV blocks, reduced respiratory rate, sweating, ataxia *Contraindications*: pre-existing cardiac dysfunction, hypotension or shock, pathological ventricular arrhythmias, respiratory dysfunction, severe hepatic or renal insufficiency, seizures.
Diltiazem	Class IV Ca^{2+}-channel blocker	0.125 mg/kg over 2 min IV, repeated every 10 min to effect, up to 1.25 mg/kg total dose	62.5 mg IV over 2 min; total dose 625 mg	Titrate to effect. Use diltiazem doses >0.5–1.0 mg/kg with caution. *Adverse effects*: hypotension, tachycardia, sinus arrhythmia, bradycardia, sinus arrest, high-grade AV block, negative inotropism, exacerbation of heart failure (unless secondary to SVT or AF with rapid ventricular response). *Contraindications*: hypotension, bradycardia, SA or AV block, ventricular systolic dysfunction, severe heart failure, cardiogenic shock, β-blockers.
First-line medication for longer-duration *rate* control				
Digoxin	Digitalis glycosides	0.0022 mg/kg every 12 h IV; 0.011 mg/kg every 12 h PO	1.1 mg IV; 5.5 mg PO	*Therapeutic drug monitoring*: peak (1–2 h) and trough (12 h) concentrations at steady state should fall within 0.8–2.0 ng/ml (1–2.6 nmol/l). *Adverse effects*: depression, anorexia, colic, diarrhoea, sinus bradycardia, AV block, supraventricular and ventricular arrhythmias (bigeminy). *Contraindications*: AV block, diastolic ventricular dysfunction, pre-existing digitalis toxicity, myocarditis, ventricular arrhythmias.

Continued

Table 5.1. Continued.

Drug	Drug class	Dose recommendations	Dose for 500 kg bwt	Comments
Sotalol	Class II/III K^+ channel and β-blocker	1 mg/kg bwt PO every 12 h for 1 day; continue at 2–3 mg/kg bwt PO every 12 h	500 mg initial dose; 1–1.5 g per maintenance dose	Good oral bioavailability. Generally well tolerated, even with chronic oral administration. Dosage should be gradually reduced before discontinuing medication. *Adverse effects*: QT prolongation, ventricular arrhythmias. *Contraindications*: pre-existing QT prolongation. Use with caution in patients with uncorrected hypokalaemia or hypomagnesaemia.
Propranolol	Class II $β_1$/ $β_2$-blocker	0.38–0.78 mg/kg bwt PO every 8 h	190–390 mg per dose	Variable bioavailability; dosage should be adjusted on an individual basis. *Adverse effects*: depression, lethargy, weakness, bradycardia, AV block, hypotension, negative inotropism, exacerbation of heart failure, bronchoconstriction (aggravation of recurrent airway obstruction). *Contraindications*: bradycardia, high-degree AV block, untreated heart failure, bronchopulmonary disease.

AF, atrial fibrillation; AV, atrioventricular; bwt, body weight; CRI, continuous rate infusion; GI, gastrointestinal; IV, intravenous; NGT, nasogastric tube; PO, per os; SA, sinoatrial; SVT, supraventricular tachycardia; VF, ventricular fibrillation; VT, ventricular tachycardia.

Table 5.2. Anti-arrhythmic drugs for use with sustained ventricular tachycardia.

Drug	Drug class	Dose recommendations	Dose for 500 kg bwt	Comments
First-line medications for *rhythm* control (IV)				
Lidocaine (lignocaine)	Class I$_B$ Na$^+$-channel blocker	0.25–0.5 mg/kg bwt slow IV, repeat in 5–10 min to effect, up to 1.5 mg/kg bwt total dose, followed by 0.05 mg/kg bwt/min CRI	125–250 mg per bolus up to total dose of 750 mg; CRI 25 mg/min	*Adverse effects*: uncommon at therapeutic doses. Overdose can lead to ataxia, muscle tremors, CNS excitement, arrhythmias and collapse. *Contraindications*: SA, AV or intraventricular block, bradycardia. Caution with hypovolaemia, liver disease, shock and heart failure.
Magnesium sulfate	Physiological Ca^{2+}- and K$^+$-channel blocker; activator of membrane Na$^+$/K$^+$-ATPase	2–6 mg/kg bwt/min IV to effect, up to 55–100 mg/kg bwt total dose	1–3 g/min; total dose 27–50 g	*Adverse effects*: rare, but overdose may lead to CNS depressant effects, weakness, trembling, bradycardia, hypotension. Very high doses cause neuromuscular blockade with respiratory depression and cardiac arrest. *Contraindications*: bradycardia, SA and AV block, renal failure.
Second-line medications for *rhythm* control (IV)				
Procainamide	Class I$_A$ Na$^+$-channel blocker	1 mg/kg bwt/min IV, up to 20 mg/kg bwt total dose	500 mg/min; total dose 10 g	*Adverse events*: hypotension, QRS and QT prolongation, negative inotropism, arrhythmia, GI and neurological disorders (similar to but generally less severe than quinidine). *Contraindications*: untreated heart failure, prolonged QRS or QT interval, complete AV block, digitalis intoxication. Use with caution in patients with hypokalaemia, hypomagnesaemia or acid–base disorders.

Continued

Table 5.2. Continued.

Drug	Drug class	Dose recommendations	Dose for 500 kg bwt	Comments
Amiodarone	Class III K$^+$-channel blocker	5 mg/kg bwt/h IV for 1 h, followed by 0.83 mg/kg bwt/h for 23 h; subsequently, 1.9 mg/kg bwt/h for 30 h or to effect	2.5 g for first hour, then 415 mg/h for the next 23 h, then 950 mg/h for additional 30 h	Also class I, II and IV effects. *Adverse reactions*: hind limb weakness, weight shifting, torsade de pointes, SA and AV nodal inhibition, bradycardia, hypotension. Prolonged treatment may affect lungs, liver, heart, thyroid gland, GI tract, eyes, skin and nerves. *Contraindications*: SA node dysfunction, bradycardia, AV block, cardiogenic shock.
Propafenone	Class I$_C$ Na$^+$-channel blocker	0.5–1.0 mg/kg bwt in 5% dextrose slow IV over 5–10 min	250–500 mg IV over 5–10 min	Not commonly available. *Adverse effects*: GI and neurological disorders, bronchospasm, negative inotropism, exacerbation of heart failure, AV block, QRS and QT prolongation, arrhythmias. *Contraindications*: structural heart disease, heart failure, SA or AV node dysfunction.
Quinidine gluconate	Class I$_A$ Na$^+$-channel blocker	1–2.2 mg/kg bwt IV every 10 min or 0.1–0.22 mg/kg bwt/min CRI up to 12 mg/kg bwt total dose	500 mg–1.1 g every 10 min or 50–110 mg/min CRI; total dose 6 g	**Use with caution.** *Adverse effects*: commonly, depression, diarrhoea, colic, ataxia, nasal mucosal swelling; less commonly, paraphimosis, urticaria, laminitis. Monitor for: Acceleration of AV conduction, tachycardia, QRS and QT prolongation, VT, torsade de pointes, hypotension, negative inotropism, exacerbation of heart failure, cardiovascular collapse, sudden death.

Continued

Table 5.2. Continued.

Drug	Drug class	Dose recommendations	Dose for 500 kg bwt	Comments
Quinidine gluconate *continued*				*Contraindications*: ventricular tachyarrhythmias, torsade de pointes, untreated heart failure, pre-existing QRS or QT interval prolongation, complete AV block, digitalis intoxication. Use with caution in patients with hypokalaemia, hypomagnesaemia, hypoxia or acid–base disorders.
Bretylium tosylate	Class III K$^+$-channel blocker	3–5 mg/kg bwt IV, repeat up to 10 mg/kg bwt total dose	1.5–2.5 g per dose; total dose 5 g	Difficult to obtain. Use in cases of refractory life-threatening VT/VF. Also has indirect anti-adrenergic effects. *Adverse effects*: excitement, GI disorders, hypotension, tachycardia, arrhythmias. *Contraindications*: pre-existing hypotension.

Second-line medications for *rhythm* control (PO)

Drug	Drug class	Dose recommendations	Dose for 500 kg bwt	Comments
Sotalol	Class II/III K$^+$-channel and β-blocker	1 mg/kg bwt PO every 12 h for 1 day; continue at 2–3 mg/kg bwt PO every 12 h	500 mg initial dose; 1–1.5 g per maintenance dose	Good oral bioavailability. Generally well tolerated, even with chronic oral administration. Dosage should be gradually reduced before discontinuing medication. *Adverse effects*: QT prolongation, ventricular arrhythmias. *Contraindications*: pre-existing QT prolongation. Use with caution in patients with uncorrected hypokalaemia or hypomagnesaemia.

Continued

Table 5.2. Continued.

Drug	Drug class	Dose recommendations	Dose for 500 kg bwt	Comments
Phenytoin	Class I_B Na$^+$-channel blocker	20 mg/kg bwt PO every 12 h for three to four doses or until signs of sedation, followed by 10–15 mg/kg bwt PO every 12 h maintenance dose	10 g loading dose; 5–7.5 g per maintenance dose	Maintenance dose varies among horses. *Therapeutic drug monitoring*: 5–10 µg/ml. *Adverse effects*: sedation, lip and facial twitching, gait deficits, excitation, seizures, arrhythmias; hepatotoxicity with chronic use. *Contraindications*: SA or AV block, sinus bradycardia.
Propafenone	Class I_C Na$^+$-channel blocker	2 mg/kg bwt PO every 8 h	1 g per dose	See adverse effects and contraindications for propafenone provided above in table.
Propranolol	Class II β_1/β_2-blocker	0.38–0.78 mg/kg bwt PO every 8 h	190–390 mg per dose	Variable bioavailability; dosage should be adjusted on an individual basis. *Adverse effects*: depression, lethargy, weakness, bradycardia, AV block, hypotension, negative inotropism, exacerbation of heart failure, bronchoconstriction (aggravation of recurrent airway obstruction). *Contraindications*: bradycardia, high-degree AV block, untreated heart failure, bronchopulmonary disease.

Continued

Table 5.2. Continued.

Drug	Drug class	Dose recommendations	Dose for 500 kg bwt	Comments
Quinidine sulfate	Class I$_A$ Na$^+$-channel blocker	22 mg/kg bwt PO by NGT every 2 h for four (up to six) doses until converted, or adverse or toxic effects, or plasma quinidine concentration >4 µg/ml. Do not exceed six doses PO within the first 12 hours.	11 g per dose	**Use with caution.** See adverse effects and contraindications provided for quinidine gluconate above in the table.

AV, atrioventricular; bwt, Body weight; CNS, central nervous system; CRI, continuous rate infusion; GI, gastrointestinal; IV, intravenous; NGT, nasogastric tube; PO, per os; SA, sinoatrial; VF, ventricular fibrillation; VT, ventricular tachycardia.

Table 5.3. Anti-arrhythmic drugs for use with intermittent arrhythmias.

Drug	Drug class	Dose recommendations	Dose for 500 kg bwt	Comments
Isolated, frequent, ventricular premature complexes:				
Consider and address primary cause (electrolyte abnormalities, myocardial disease, toxins, SIRS) before initiating anti-arrhythmic therapy				
Sotalol	Class II/III K$^+$-channel and β-blocker	1 mg/kg bwt PO every 12 h for 1 day, continue at 2–3 mg/kg bwt PO every 12 h	500 mg initial dose; 1–1.5 g per maintenance dose	Good oral bioavailability. Generally well tolerated, even with chronic oral administration. Dosage should be gradually reduced before discontinuing medication. *Adverse effects*: QT prolongation, ventricular arrhythmias. *Contraindications*: pre-existing QT prolongation. Use with caution in patients with uncorrected hypokalaemia or hypomagnesaemia.
Phenytoin	Class I$_B$ Na$^+$-channel blocker	20 mg/kg bwt PO every 12 h for three to four doses or until signs of sedation, followed by 10–15 mg/kg bwt PO every 12 h per maintenance dose	10 g loading dose; 5–7.5 g per maintenance dose	Maintenance dose varies among horses. *Therapeutic drug monitoring*: 5–10 μg/ml. *Adverse effects*: sedation, lip and facial twitching, gait deficits, excitation, seizures, arrhythmias; hepatotoxicity with chronic use. *Contraindications*: SA or AV block, sinus bradycardia.

Continued

Table 5.3. Continued.

Drug	Drug class	Dose recommendations	Dose for 500 kg bwt	Comments
Isolated, frequent, atrial premature complexes:				
Consider and address primary cause (electrolyte abnormalities, myocardial disease, toxins, SIRS) before initiating anti-arrhythmic therapy				
Sotalol	Class II/III K$^+$-channel and β-blocker	1 mg/kg bwt PO every 12 h for 1 day; continue at 2–3 mg/ kg bwt PO every 12 h	500 mg initial dose; 1–1.5 g per maintenance dose	Good oral bioavailability. Generally well tolerated, even with chronic oral administration. Dosage should be gradually reduced before discontinuing medication. *Adverse effects*: QT prolongation, ventricular arrhythmias. *Contraindications*: pre-existing QT prolongation. Use with caution in patients with uncorrected hypokalaemia or hypomagnesaemia.

AV, atrioventricular; bwt, body weight; PO, per os; SA, sinoatrial; SIRS, systemic inflammatory response syndrome.

Table 5.4. Pharmacological evaluation of bradyarrhythmias.

Drug	Drug class	Dose recommendations	Dose for 500 kg bwt	Comments
Bradyarrhythmias causing hypotension (sinus arrest, sinus bradycardia, high-grade or complete AV block): **These medications should be used to provide confirmation of the arrhythmia (based on a failure to respond appropriately to the medication) and to provide temporary therapy until a longer-term solution can be found (i.e. pacemaker implantation)**				
Dopamine	β_1-adrenergic, dose-dependent dopaminergic and α_1-adrenergic	1–5 µg/kg bwt/min CRI, titrate to effect or adverse reaction	500–2500 µg/min CRI	*Adverse effects*: tachycardia, ventricular arrhythmias, vasoconstriction and hypertension (at doses >4 µg/kg bwt/min).
Dobutamine	β_1-adrenergic, β_2- and α_1-adrenergic; preferred over dopamine	1–5 µg/kg bwt/min CRI, titrate to effect or adverse reaction	500–2500 µg/min CRI	*Contraindications*: ventricular arrhythmias, tachycardia, atrial fibrillation (risk of severe tachycardia due to accelerated AV conduction).
Atropine	Anticholinergic (vagolytic)	0.01–0.02 mg/kg bwt IV or IM	5–10 mg IV or IM	*Adverse effects*: constipation, ileus, colic, bradycardia (at very low doses), tachycardia, arrhythmias, CNS effects (stimulation, drowsiness, ataxia, seizures, respiratory depression). Glycopyrrolate is slightly less arrhythmogenic and rarely results in CNS effects.
Glycopyrrolate	Anticholinergic (vagolytic)	0.005–0.01 mg/kg bwt IV	2.5–5 mg IV	*Contraindications*: tachycardia, tachyarrhythmia, heart failure, GI disease, colic.

AV, atrioventricular; bwt, body weight; CNS, central nervous system; CRI, continuous rate infusion; GI, gastrointestinal; IM, intramuscular; IV, intravenous.

Assessment of Risk and Safety

In equine practice, we are frequently asked to assess the risk of an adverse event occurring, both at rest and during exercise but particularly when exercising at high speed, over obstacles or in difficult terrain, where the consequences of an adverse event are particularly life-threatening.

It is clear that sustained arrhythmias occurring at rapid heart rates will be haemodynamically relevant, leading to weakness, stumbling and, in severe cases, collapse or sudden death. It can be more difficult to estimate the potential haemodynamic effects of sustained arrhythmias occurring at lower heart rates, or arrhythmias only occurring intermittently. Here, other individual factors, including any concurrent disease, stress, fatigue, exercise or rider experience will influence the consequences of any arrhythmia present.

From the perspective of ECG interpretation and diagnoses, the assessment of safety and risk can be divided into several categories, as seen in Box 6.1.

The ECG findings should always be interpreted together with the clinical examination, any findings on haematology or chemistry evaluation, and in conjunction with the echocardiographic information. The presence of underlying structural heart disease (e.g. cardiac chamber enlargement, myocardial hypertrophy or myocardial echogenicity) in combination with arrhythmia is considered to increase the risk of an adverse event.

In horses with a history of collapse, even if no clear cause of collapse is identified on examination, these horses should be considered at higher risk of a future adverse event compared with healthy horses.

Box 6.1. Stratification of risk of arrhythmia on safety.

- **Sustained arrhythmias that pose an immediate threat to life:**
  - Ventricular flutter/ fibrillation
  - Polymorphic ventricular tachycardia
  - Torsade de pointes
  - R-on-T phenomenon.
- **Sustained arrhythmias that can cause morbidity and, without treatment, can become life threatening:**
  - Monomorphic ventricular tachycardia
  - Rapid supraventricular tachycardia (rate >120 bpm)
  - Accelerated idioventricular/junctional rhythms (particularly when myocardial dysfunction is present or if they deteriorate to ventricular tachycardia)
  - Third-degree (complete) atrioventricular block.
- **Sustained arrhythmias that are usually well tolerated at rest but can impact performance and have the potential to become life threatening:**
  - Supraventricular tachycardia (e.g. atrial fibrillation)
  - Accelerated idio-ventricular/junctional rhythms
  - High-grade second-degree AV block (particularly if deteriorating to third-degree AV block)
  - High-grade sinus block, sinus arrest or profound sinus bradycardia.
- **Intermittent arrhythmias occurring at rest or during exercise that can impact performance and have the potential to become life threatening:**
  - Frequent ventricular premature complexes, couplets, triplets and short runs of ventricular tachycardia, particularly when R-on-T phenomenon is present.
- **Intermittent arrhythmias occurring at rest or during exercise that may become performance limiting but are unlikely to become life threatening:**
  - Frequent atrial premature complexes, couplets or triplets, and short runs of supraventricular tachycardia with longer coupling intervals.

ECG Interpretation in Pre-purchase Examinations

Arrhythmias are detected frequently during pre-purchase examinations, particularly after exercise. It can be difficult to differentiate between normal physiological arrhythmias and those with pathological consequences on auscultation alone.

During a pre-purchase examination, it can be helpful to confirm the presence of a normal sinus rhythm with a short ECG recording. This can be obtained quickly with a hand-held device such as the AliveCor KardiaMobile ECG Monitor (AliveCor, Mountain View, California, USA).

If an arrhythmia is heard, an ECG recording should be obtained to diagnose the type of arrhythmia. In performance horses with arrhythmias, an exercising ECG (including the recovery phase) should also be recorded and analysed.

The recommendations for horses with arrhythmias heard on pre-purchase examination are described in Box 7.1.

Box 7.1. Recommendations for horses with arrhythmias heard on pre-purchase examination. (Information from Reef, 2019; Reef *et al.*, 2014.)

- **Horses with high-grade second-degree atrioventricular (AV) block, sinus block, sinus arrest or profound sinus bradycardia:**
  - Even if these rhythms are overdriven with stress or exercise, the horse is not considered suitable for a child rider, for hire or when used in a lesson programme
  - They should only be exercised by an informed adult
  - There is a risk of a high-grade second-degree AV block progressing to a third-degree (complete) AV block.
- **Horses with atrial premature complexes or ventricular premature complexes:**
  - Occasional atrial premature complexes (APCs) that are overdriven by stress or exercise or occur infrequently during exercise are considered as safe to use for performance as their age-matched peers
  - Horses with APCs may have an increased risk of developing atrial fibrillation; however, the magnitude of this risk is unknown
  - Occasional uniform ventricular premature complexes (VPCs) in horses with no evidence of underlying structural heart disease, and that are overdriven during stress or exercise, are considered suitable for an informed adult rider/driver but are not considered suitable for a child rider, for hire or for use as a lesson horse
  - Frequent or multiform VPCs, the R-on-T phenomenon or complex ventricular arrhythmias are more likely to be associated with underlying myocardial disease. These horses are considered more likely to have an adverse event (e.g. collapse or sudden death) than a healthy horse.

- **Horses with atrial fibrillation (and other supraventricular tachycardias):**
  - For horses without a history of exercise intolerance and with no evidence of underlying structural disease, an appropriate heart-rate response during exercise, without evidence of ventricular arrhythmia/aberrant conduction/R-on-T phenomenon during stress or exercise:
    - The possibilities, risks and costs of conversion from atrial fibrillation to normal sinus rhythm should be discussed with the purchaser.
    - Some horses can remain in atrial fibrillation and, depending on the type and intensity of exercise, perform to expectation. The expectations of performance should be discussed with the purchaser.
    - Horses in sustained atrial fibrillation are not considered suitable for a child rider, for hire or for use as a lesson horse. They should only be exercised by an informed adult.
  - For horses with an absence of structural heart disease but exercise intolerance, a high ventricular response rate or ventricular arrhythmias/aberrant conduction/R-on-T phenomenon:
    - These horses are considered a safety risk and are unlikely to perform at their intended level (exercise or breeding).
    - Conversion of atrial fibrillation to normal sinus rhythm is recommended and should be discussed with the purchaser, including the method, risks, costs and recurrence rates.
  - Horses with relevant underlying structural disease:
    - Conversion is not recommended.
    - These horses are considered a safety risk and are unlikely to perform at their intended level (exercise or breeding). This should be discussed with the purchaser.

- **Horses with accelerated idioventricular/junctional rhythms or history of ventricular tachycardia:**
  - There is concern about underlying myocardial disease being present in these horses. If myocardial abnormalities are detected on echocardiography, the risk of an adverse event is considered even higher
  - Even if these rhythms are overdriven with stress or exercise, the horse is not considered suitable for a child rider, for hire or for use as a lesson horse
  - These horses should only be exercised by informed adult riders.

Case Examples

Case 1

Figure 8.1 shows an ECG obtained from a horse at rest. What is the diagnosis?

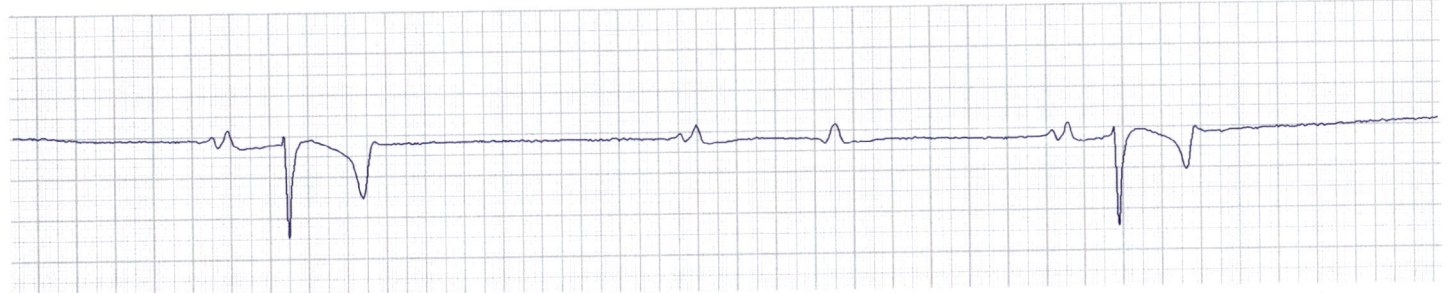

Fig. 8.1. ECG from a horse at rest. Paper speed: 50 mm/s.

Case 2

Figure 8.2 shows an ECG obtained from a horse at rest. The horse has severe aortic regurgitation with moderate left ventricular enlargement. No exercise intolerance is reported. What is the diagnosis? What are your safety recommendations for this horse?

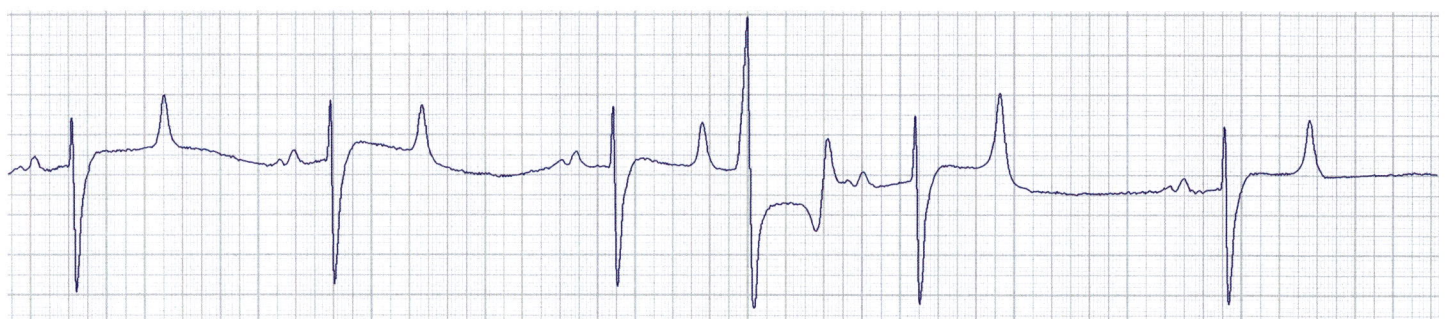

Fig. 8.2. ECG from a horse at rest. Paper speed: 50 mm/s.

Case 3

Figure 8.3 shows an ECG obtained from a horse at rest. Leads I and II are both displayed for reference. What is your diagnosis? What are your recommendations for this horse?

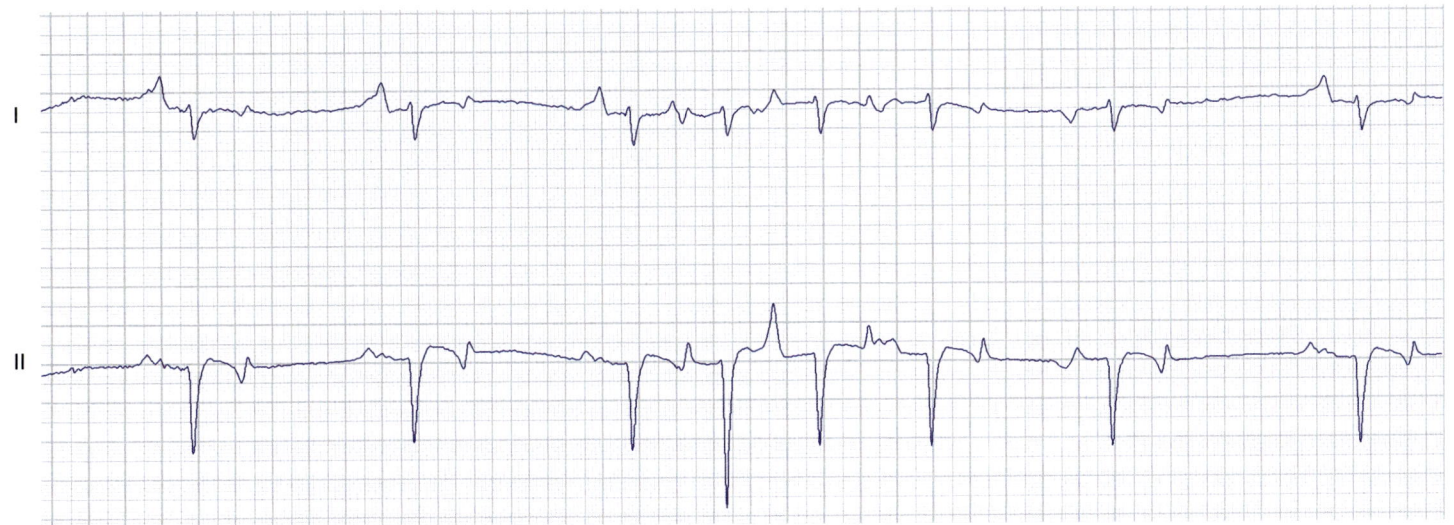

Fig. 8.3. ECG from a horse at rest. Paper speed: 50 mm/s.

Case 4

Figure 8.4 shows an ECG from a horse at rest. What is your diagnosis?

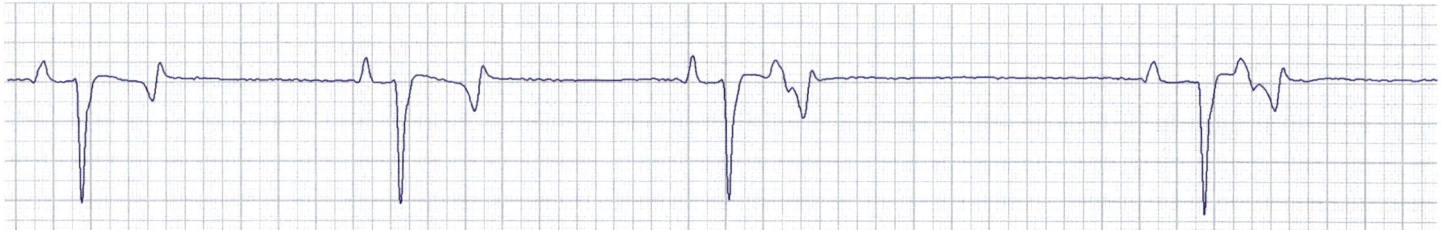

Fig. 8.4. ECG from a horse at rest. Paper speed: 50 mm/s.

Case 5

Figure 8.5 shows an ECG from a horse at rest. What is your diagnosis?

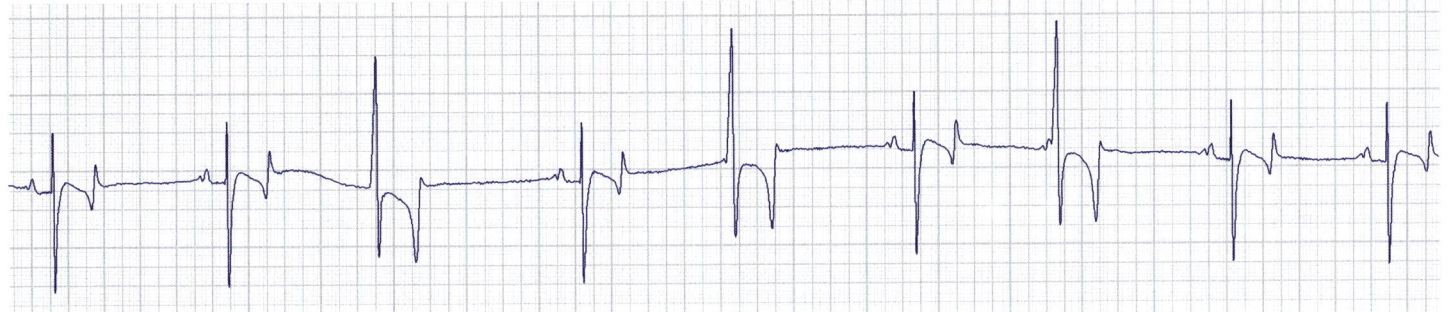

Fig. 8.5. ECG from a horse at rest. Paper speed: 25 mm/s.

Case 6

Figure 8.6, shows an ECG from a horse presented for evaluation of acute exercise intolerance and increased effort breathing. What is your diagnosis? What are your recommendations for this horse?

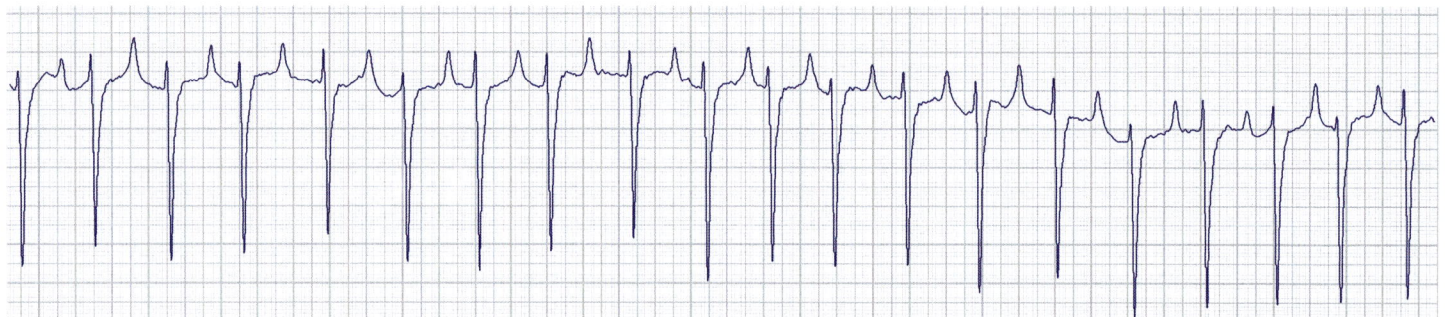

Fig. 8.6. ECG from a horse presented for evaluation of acute exercise intolerance and increased effort breathing. Paper speed: 50 mm/s.

Case 7

Figure 8.7 shows an ECG of a horse presented for evaluation of colic, sweating and anxiety. What is your diagnosis? What are your recommendations for this case?

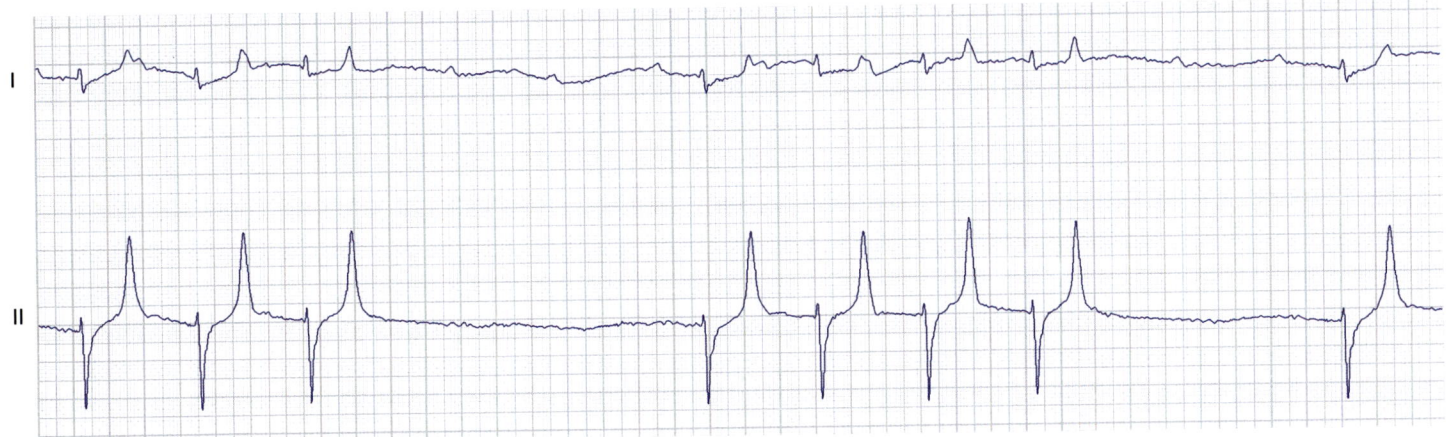

Fig. 8.7. ECG from a horse presented for evaluation of colic, sweating and anxiety. Paper speed: 50 mm/s.

Case 8

Figure 8.8 shows a resting ECG recording from a horse presented for exercise intolerance. What is your diagnosis?

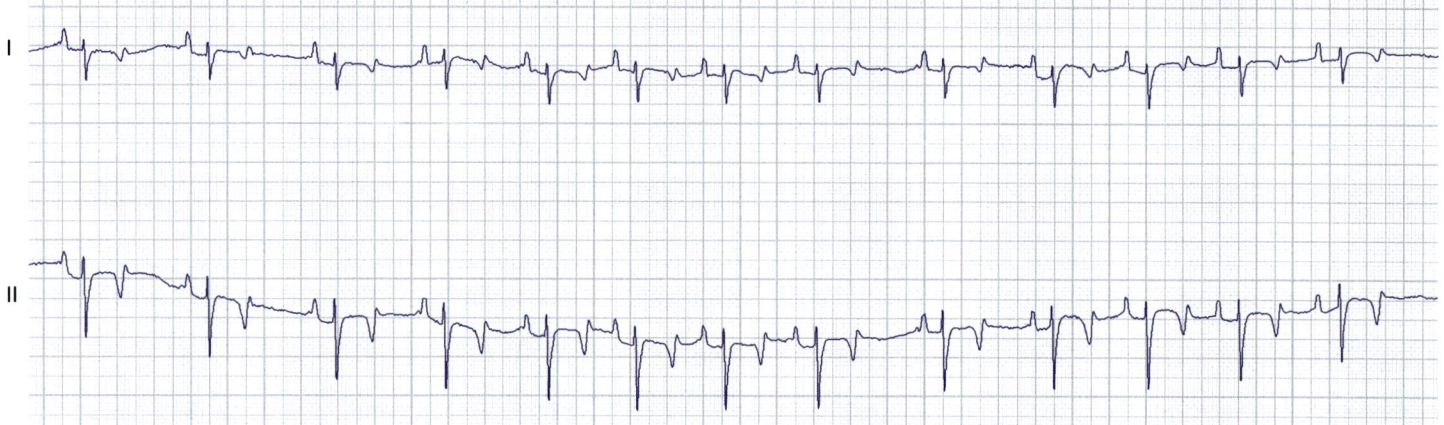

Fig. 8.8. Resting ECG from a horse presented for exercise intolerance. Paper speed: 25 mm/s.

Case 9

Figure 8.9 shows ECGs from a dressage horse with exercise intolerance. What is your diagnosis in Fig. 8.9A? What are the ECG changes in Figs. 8.9B and C? What is the cause of these changes? What are your recommendations for the management of this case?

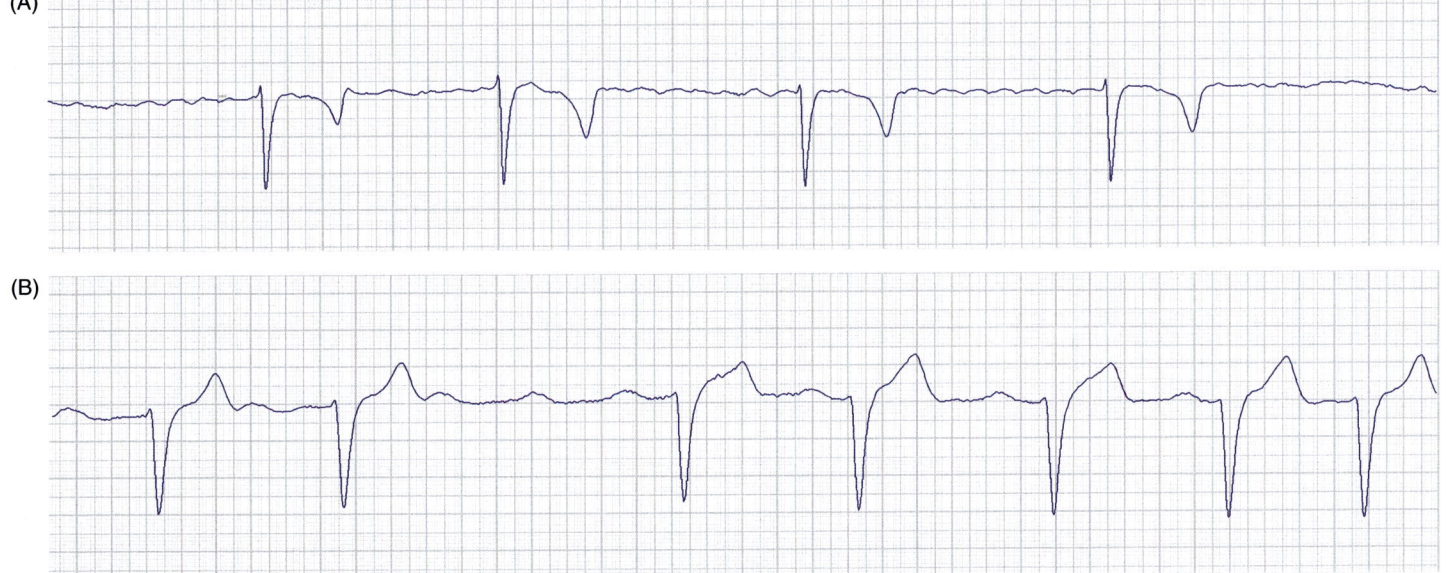

Fig. 8.9. ECGs from a dressage horse with exercise intolerance. Paper speed: 50 mm/s.

(C)

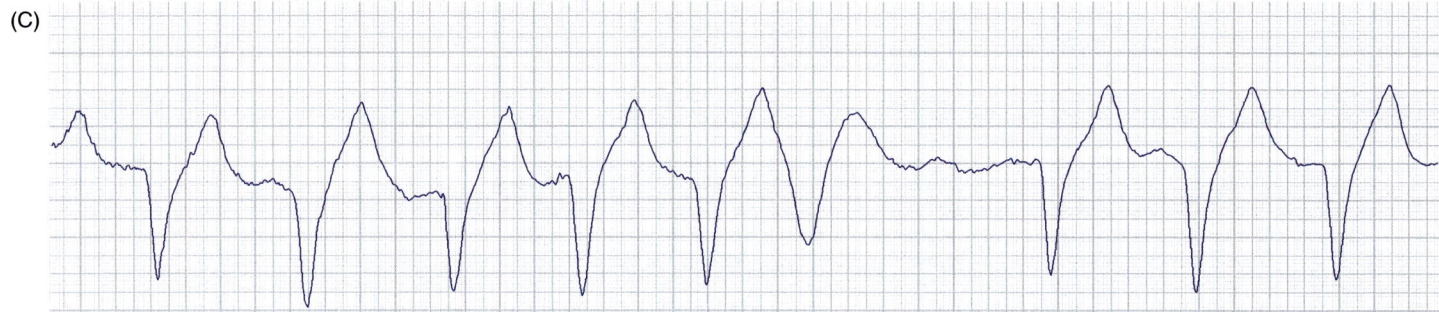

Fig. 8.9. Continued

Case 10

Figure 8.10 shows an ECG obtained using the AliveCor Kardia smartphone app. This horse was presented for oesophageal obstruction and treated for subsequent severe aspiration pneumonia. Ten days after commencing treatment, the horse was dull and inappetent, and showed fluctuations in heart rate with periods of 40–50 bpm and periods of 80–100 bpm. What is your diagnosis? What are your recommendations for management of this case?

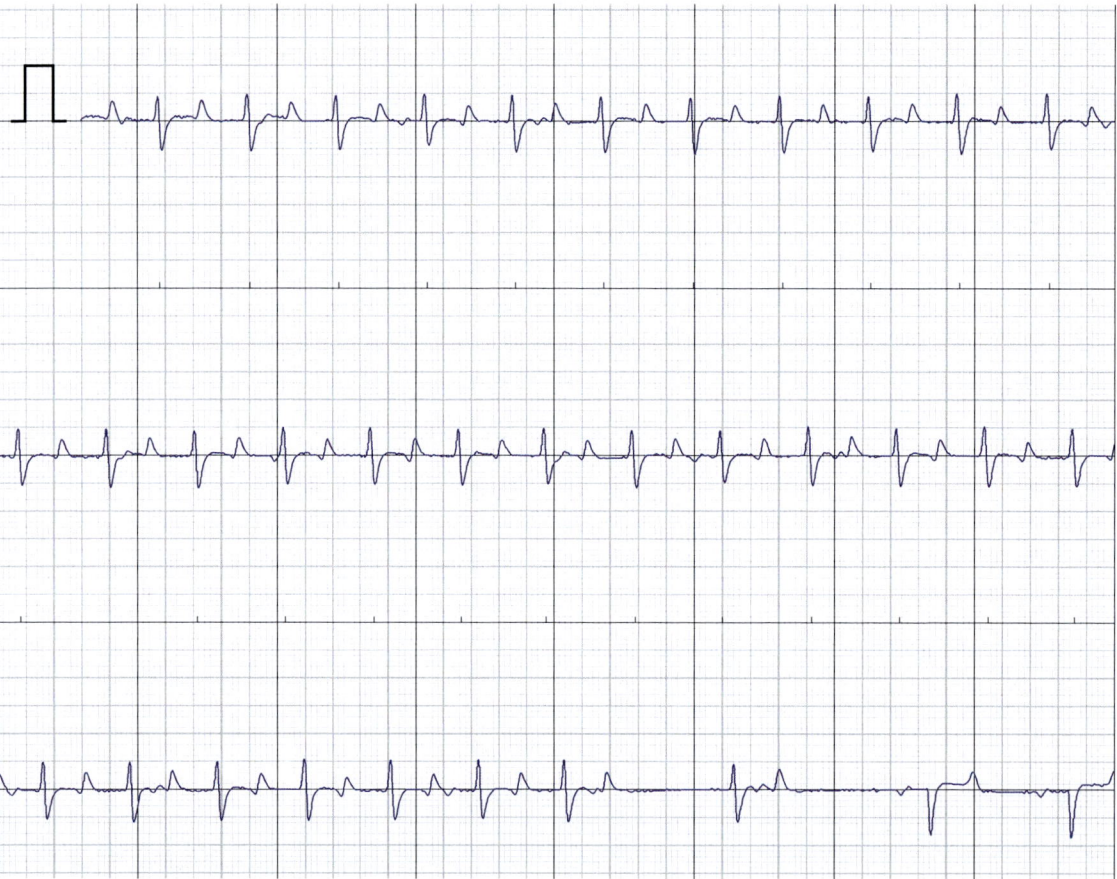

Fig. 8.10. ECG obtained using the AliveCor Kardia smartphone app. Paper speed: 25 mm/s.

Case Examples – Answers

Case 1 Answer

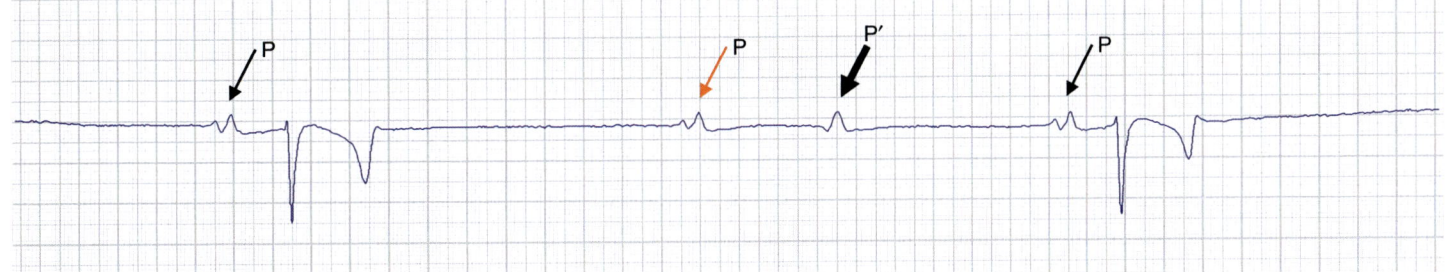

Fig. 8.1. ECG from a horse at rest. Paper speed: 50 mm/s.

There are two normal P-QRS-T complexes (black arrows) with a normal P wave that is not conducted (second-degree atrioventricular (AV) block; orange arrow) seen between the two normal complexes. Following the second-degree AV block, there is an atrial premature complex (APC, P′ wave; bold black arrow) that is not conducted to the ventricle. Note the different morphology of the P′ wave. The atrial rate is 40 bpm, while the ventricular rate is 20 bpm in this ECG segment.

Case 2 Answer

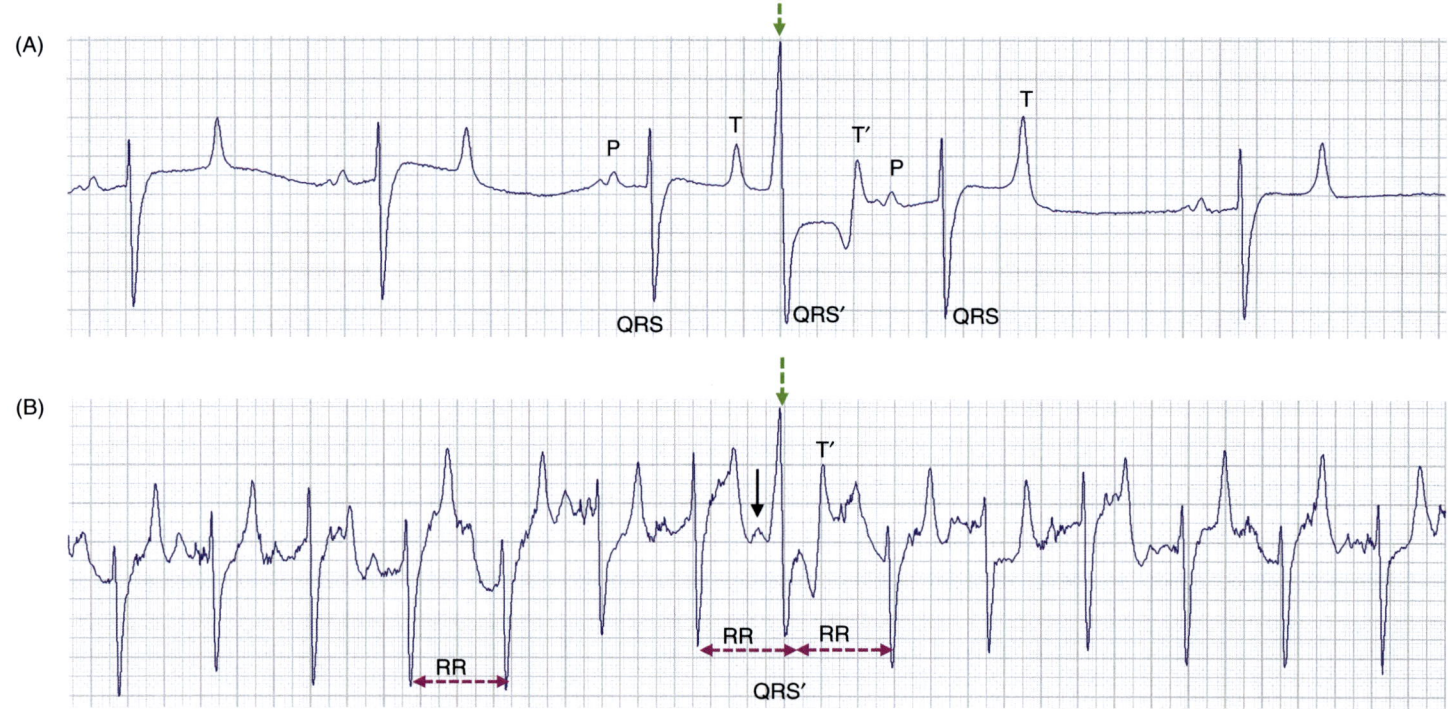

Fig. 8.2. A. ECG from a horse at rest. Paper speed: 50 mm/s. B. ECG from the same horse during exercise. Paper speed 50 mm/s.

A ventricular premature complex (VPC; green dashed arrow) is interpolated between two normal P-QRS-T complexes (Fig. 8.2A). There is no change to the underlying sinus rhythm, which continues on without a pause.

Over a 24 h period, several hundred similar-morphology VPCs were observed, occasionally in couplets and triplets. No R-on-T phenomenon was identified.

Given the underlying structural heart disease, the ventricular ectopy is considered most likely to be secondary to myocardial disease. If the horse is to be exercised, an exercising ECG should be performed. Even if the exercising ECG is normal, this horse is not considered suitable for a child rider, for hire or for use as a lesson horse. It should only be ridden by an informed adult rider/driver. This horse is considered more likely to have an adverse event (e.g. collapse or sudden death) than a healthy horse.

An exercising ECG was obtained from this horse (Fig. 8.2B). The horse was lunged for 7 min at walk, trot and canter. During this period of time, 26 VPCs were detected. An example of a VPC (green dashed arrow) is seen here, with a similar morphology to those VPCs at rest. The abnormal complex is earlier (purple double-ended arrows indicate the regular RR interval) and is followed by a pause. The encompassing RR interval is twice that of normal, indicating no change to the underlying sinus rhythm. The normal P wave (black arrow) can be seen immediately prior to the abnormal QRS complex. This PR interval is too short to be considered physiological; there is AV dissociation present.

Given these findings, this horse is considered to be at an even higher risk of an adverse event (e.g. collapse or sudden death). Exercising this horse is not recommended.

Case 3 Answer

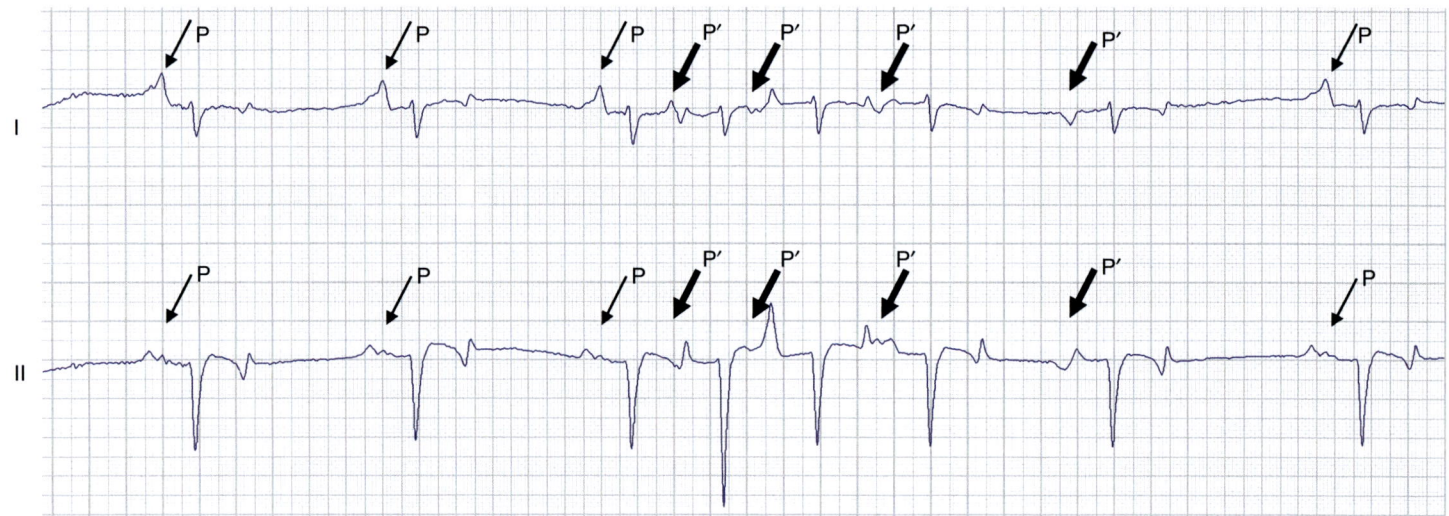

Fig. 8.3. ECG from a horse at rest. Paper speed: 50 mm/s.

A short run of atrial tachycardia is present (four APCs, bold arrows). The P′ waves have different morphology from the sinus-origin P waves. It is easier to identify the P′ waves in the recording from lead I. The first premature P′ wave is found buried in the preceding T wave, and the following QRS complex is larger with a secondary T-wave morphology change due to the short coupling interval of this premature complex with the preceding beat. The remaining QRS-T complexes are similar to the morphology of the sinus-origin beats.

    This is an ECG from a horse 48 h after transvenous electrical cardioversion of atrial fibrillation to sinus rhythm.

    APCs are considered potential triggers for atrial fibrillation. In a horse shortly after conversion from atrial fibrillation to sinus rhythm, these complexes are considered more of a risk for inducing recurrence.

    This horse was treated with the class II/III anti-arrhythmic drug sotalol. A substantial reduction in APC frequency could be seen on the 24 h ECG recording. Sotalol was continued for 1 month after conversion. At a recheck examination after 1 month, very low numbers of APCs were observed and sotalol was discontinued. The horse was still in sinus rhythm 1 year later.

Case 4 Answer

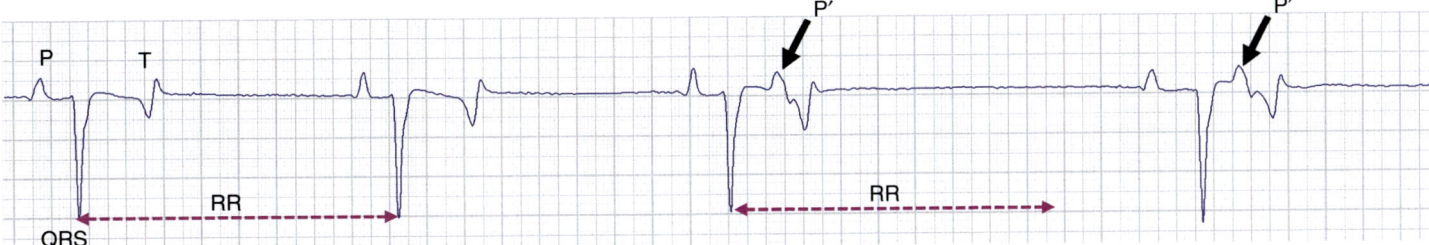

Fig. 8.4. ECG from a horse at rest. Paper speed: 50 mm/s.

Here two normal sinus-origin P-QRS-T complexes are seen on the left of the ECG. The following two complexes have APCs buried in the ST segment (P′, bold arrows). Neither of these premature complexes are conducted due to the refractoriness of the nodal and ventricular tissue. Note that the RR interval (purple double-ended arrows) is prolonged after the APC, as a result of sinoatrial node (SA) depolarization. The SA node is 'reset', which delays the next sinus complex.

If you identify pauses on an ECG tracing, it is important to evaluate the preceding QRS complex, ST segment and T wave for any hidden APCs.

APCs can trigger atrial fibrillation. Frequent APCs are abnormal findings and increase the risk of developing atrial fibrillation, particularly in a horse with a large atrial myocardial substrate.

Case 5 Answer

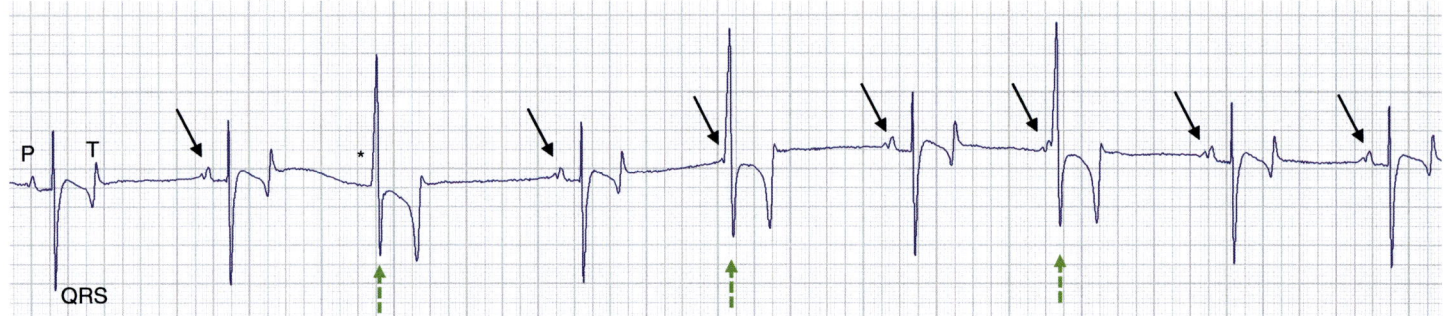

Fig. 8.5. ECG from a horse at rest. Paper speed: 25 mm/s.

This is a period of ventricular bigeminy. A normal P-QRS-T complex is followed by a VPC (green dashed arrows). The sinus-origin P waves (black arrows) can be identified within the abnormal QRS complexes. The asterisk (*) indicates that the normal P wave is superimposed on the abnormal QRS complex and is not detected. The abnormal QRS complexes show Rs morphology and have a long coupling interval with the preceding normal complex; therefore, the underlying rhythm does not appear particularly irregular.

Case 6 Answer

(A)

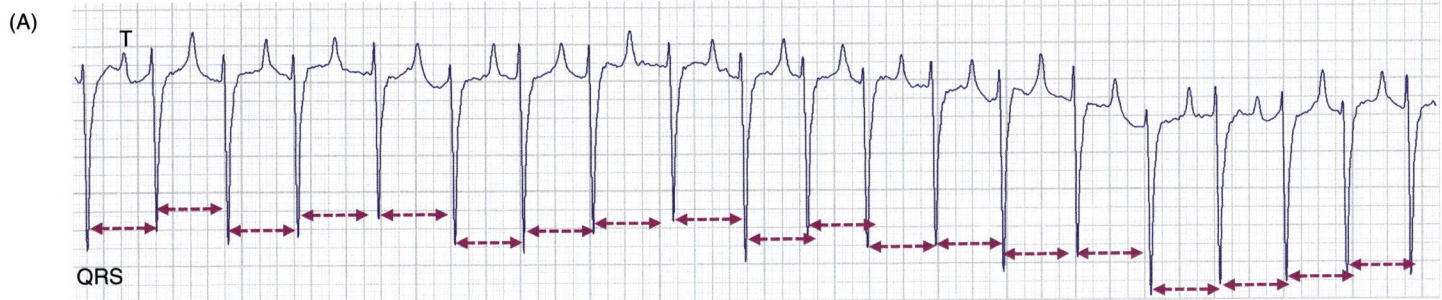

(B)

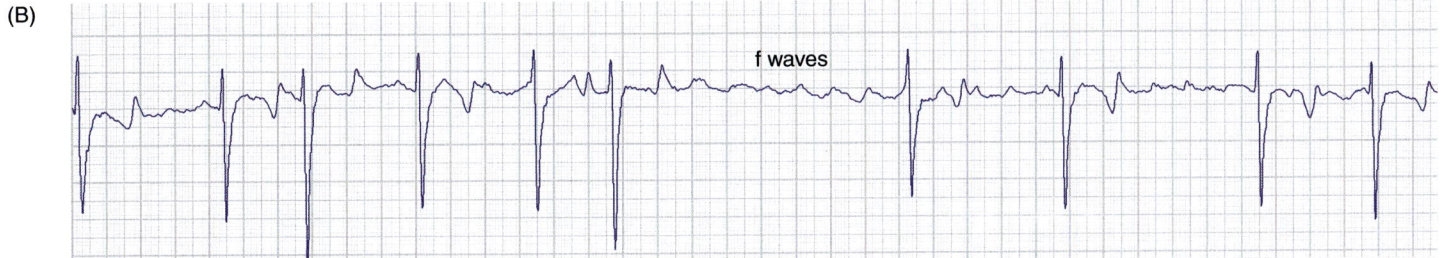

Fig. 8.6. A. ECG from a horse presented for evaluation of acute exercise intolerance and increased effort breathing. Paper speed: 50 mm/s. B. The same horse following a low dose of the alpha-2 agonist xylazine, which slowed the AV node conduction. Paper speed: 50 mm/s.

This is a supraventricular tachycardia (Fig. 8.6A). The ventricular rate is 140 bpm. The RR intervals are irregularly irregular (purple double-ended arrows indicate the first RR interval of the ECG). No clear P waves can be identified at this rate, so it is difficult to differentiate between atrial tachycardia, atrial flutter and atrial fibrillation as the underlying rhythm. The QRS morphology appears narrow and of normal polarity, and the T waves are of normal size.

At this rapid ventricular rate, the rhythm is becoming haemodynamically relevant, resulting in the clinical signs of exercise intolerance and increased respiratory rate.

The horse should be stabilized with intravenous (IV) fluids to improve cardiac output and kept as calm as possible to reduce sympathetic stimulation. In this case, a low dose of xylazine was given slowly (0.3 mg/kg IV, over 2–3 min) to try and block the rapid ventricular conduction for a short period of time. This resulted in the ECG seen in Fig. 8.6B. Here, the ventricular response has slowed to 70 bpm. In the pauses between QRS complexes, irregular fibrillation (f) waves can be detected, while the rhythm remains irregularly irregular. This confirms that the underlying rhythm is atrial fibrillation, with a rapid ventricular response.

In this horse, when the rapid ventricular conduction was present, myocardial function was abnormal with a severely shortened ventricular filling time during diastole (seen on echocardiography). Attempts to gain longer-term control of the ventricular response rate with digoxin (0.0022 mg/kg IV every 12 h for 24 h, followed by 0.011 mg/kg PO every 12 h for 6 days) was unsuccessful at reducing the ventricular rate to normal values, although the ventricular rate dropped below 100 bpm and the horse was clinically stable.

Echocardiography performed at lower heart rates (ventricular rate 70–90 bpm) with the horse haemodynamically stable did not reveal underlying structural heart disease that would preclude an attempt at cardioversion. Therefore, after 7 days of therapy, transvenous electrical cardioversion was performed. The horse converted to sinus rhythm on the second shock of 125 J. He recovered uneventfully and was still in sinus rhythm 2 years later. His exercise intolerance resolved immediately after conversion.

This is an example of atrial fibrillation with a rapid ventricular response, which is less commonly reported in horses compared with other species. There was no evidence of underlying structural heart disease, or evidence of an accessory pathway that could explain the rapid ventricular conduction. In this case, the rapid response was probably related to vagosympathetic balance, with an increase in sympathetic tone and decrease in vagal tonic inhibition.

Case 7 Answer

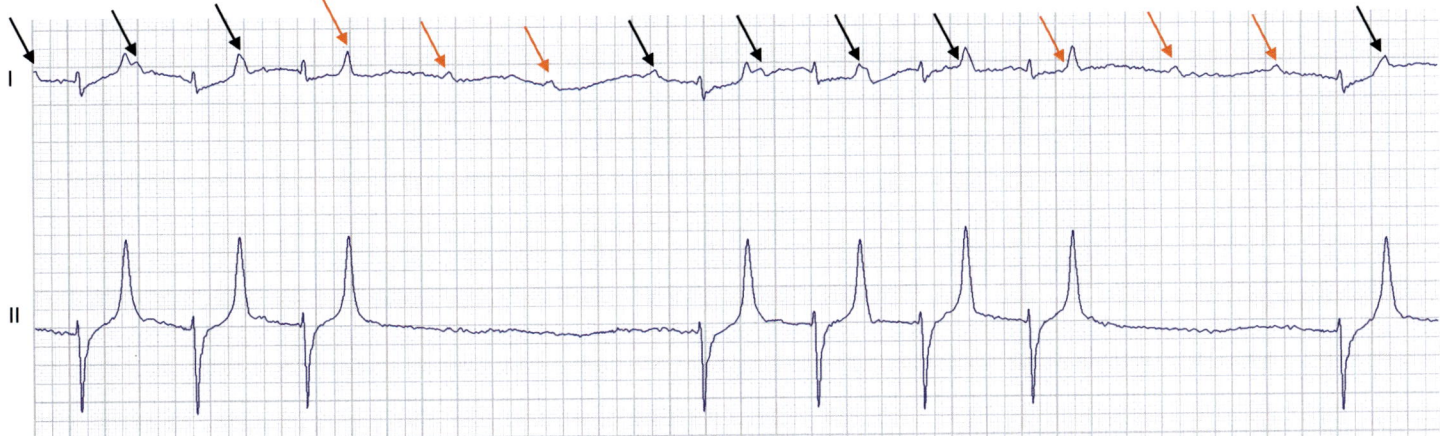

Fig. 8.7. ECG from a horse presented for evaluation of colic, sweating and anxiety. Paper speed: 50 mm/s.

This is a sinus tachycardia with high-grade second-degree AV blocks (black arrows indicate conducted P waves, orange arrows indicate P waves that were not conducted). The atrial rate is 110 bpm, while the ventricular rate is 70 bpm. The QRS morphology is normal; however, the T waves are relatively large, probably due to the rapid rate and underlying disease. The P waves are more easily identified in the tracing from lead I. Given the rapid heart rate, these second-degree AV blocks are considered pathological.

It is important to measure the blood pressure in cases where second-degree AV blocks are found at higher heart rates. In cases of hypertension, the baroreceptor reflex will increase vagal tone (delaying AV nodal conduction) to try to control the blood pressure through heart rate reduction.

The blood pressure (measured non-invasively from the coccygeal artery) revealed a systolic blood pressure of 215 mmHg, diastolic blood pressure of 116 mmHg and a mean arterial pressure of 148 mmHg.

Causes of systemic hypertension in horses include stress, exercise, renal disease and pain. In this case, the combination of colic signs, extreme anxiety and sweating combined with hypertension was caused by a phaeochromocytoma. This horse had a number of arrhythmias detected on the 24 h ECG recording, including paroxysmal atrial fibrillation, sinus tachycardia, high-grade second-degree AV blocks and ventricular tachycardia. In horses with phaeochromocytoma, arrhythmias are a common finding. This can be due to the combination of excessive catecholamine production inducing arrhythmias, myocardial hypoxia resulting from profound vasoconstriction and myocardial hypertrophy secondary to the systemic hypertension.

Case 8 Answer

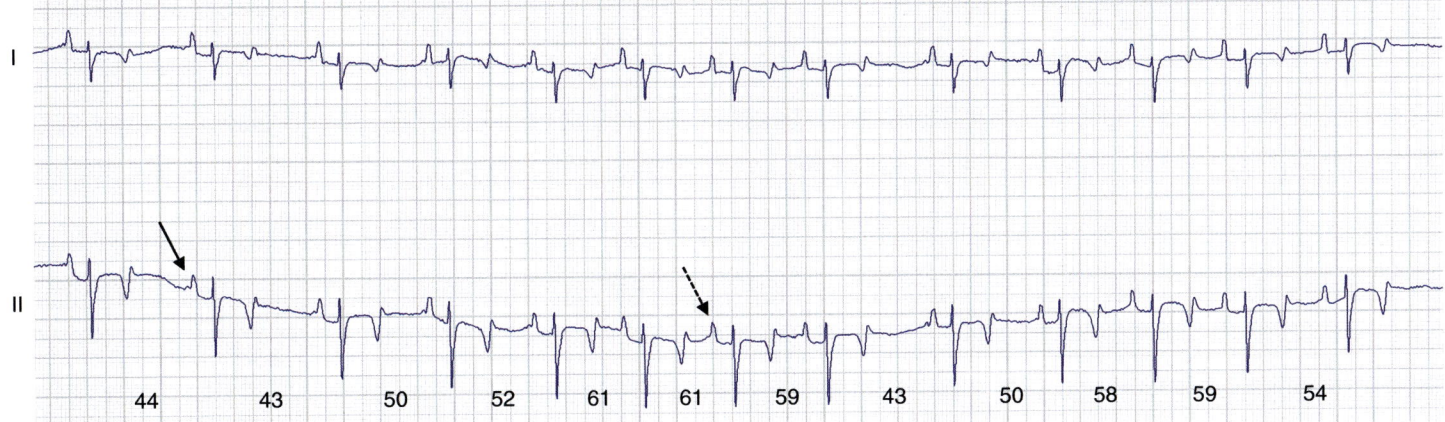

Fig. 8.8. Resting ECG from a horse presented for exercise intolerance. The sinus rate is shown below the trace. Paper speed: 25 mm/s.

This is a sinus arrhythmia. The sinus rate can be seen speeding up and slowing down. With sinus arrhythmia, the decelerations are often a little more abrupt than the heart rate accelerations. As the rate increases, the P waves become larger and monophasic (dashed arrow), while at lower rates they have a bifid appearance (solid arrow). The QRS-T complexes have a normal appearance.

In this case, the 24 h and exercising ECGs did not reveal any pathological abnormalities. The horse was diagnosed with moderate equine asthma, explaining the exercise intolerance.

Case 9 Answer

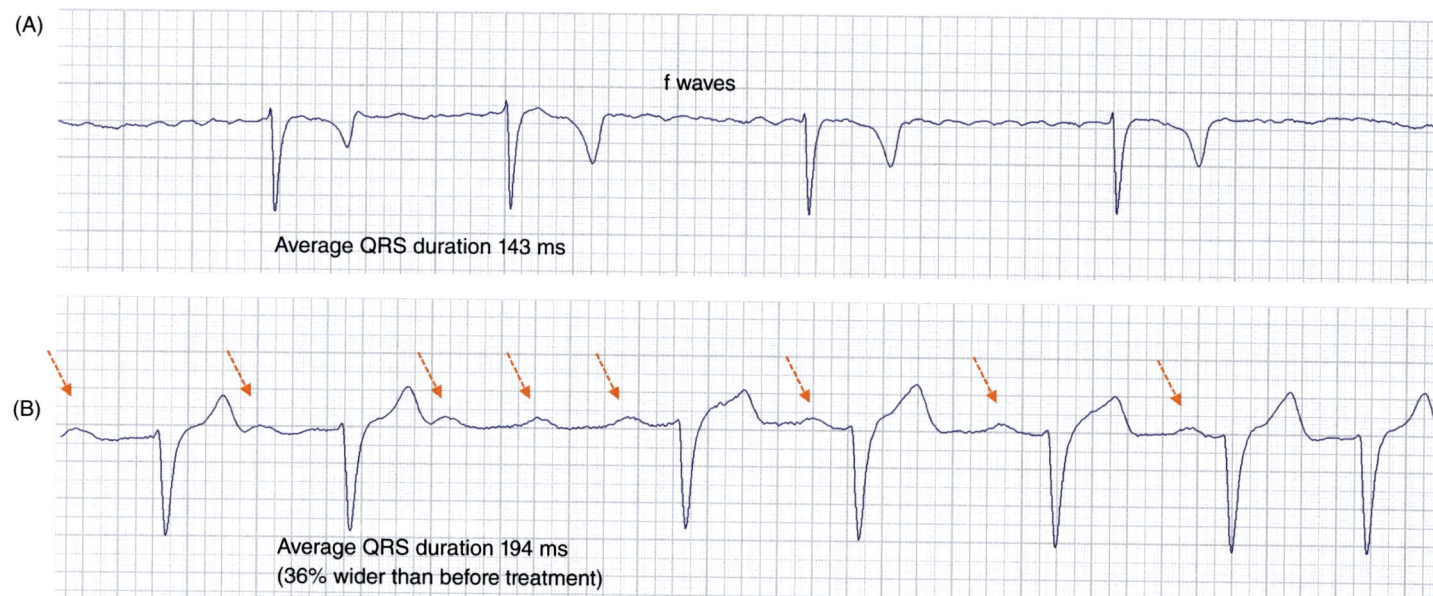

Fig. 8.9. A. ECGs from a dressage horse with exercise intolerance. Paper speed: 50 mm/s. B. ECG from the same horse during quinidine sulfate therapy in an attempt to convert the atrial fibrillation to sinus rhythm. Paper speed: 50 mm/s.

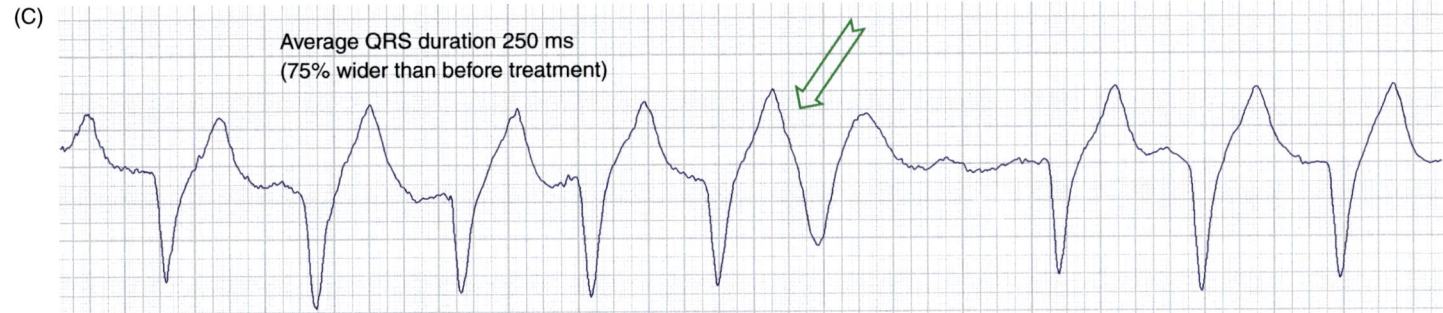

(C)

Average QRS duration 250 ms
(75% wider than before treatment)

Fig. 8.9. Continued C. ECG from the same horse, 1.5 hours after the 8th dose of quinidine sulfate. Paper speed 50 mm/s.

(D)

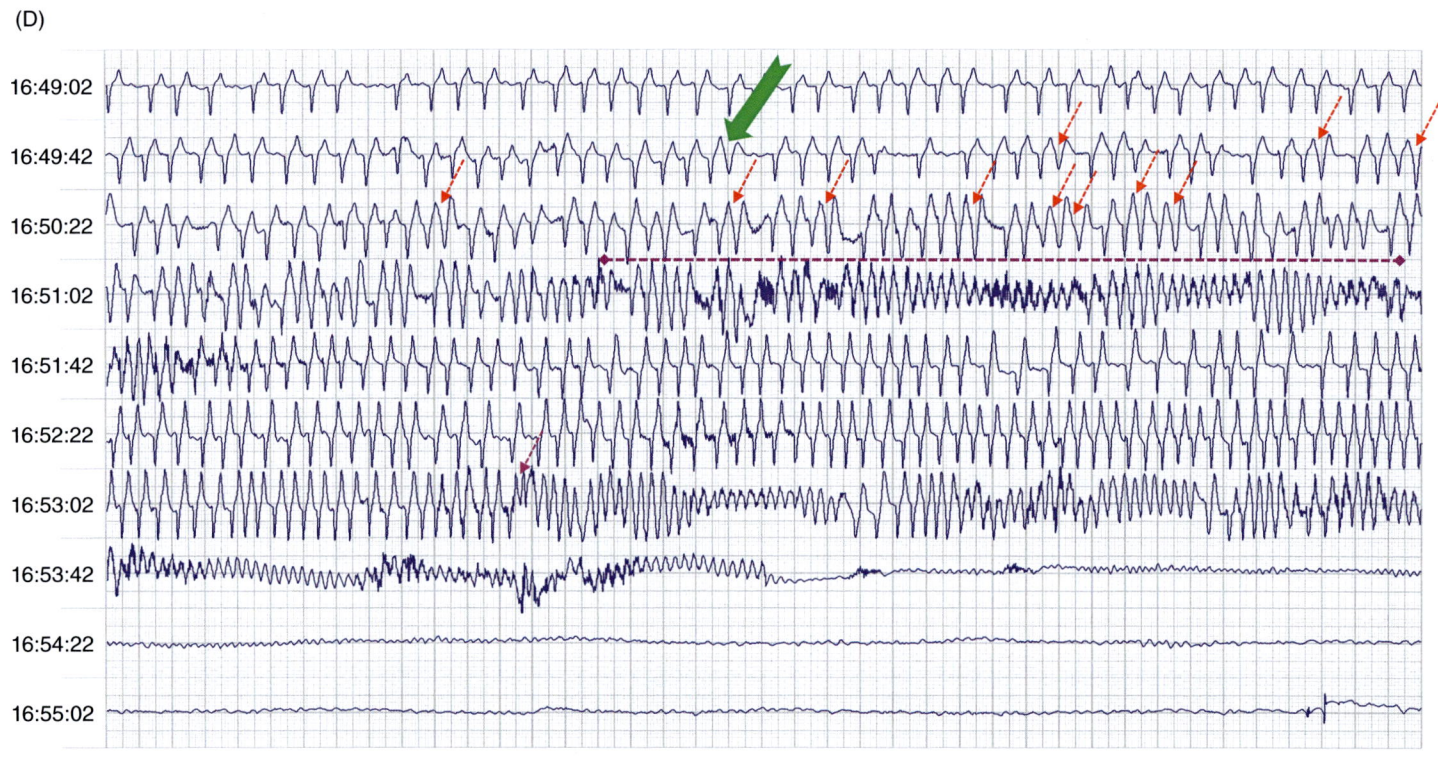

Fig. 8.9. Continued D. Overview of the rhythm leading up to the collapse and sudden death of this horse.

The ECG in Fig. 8.9A shows atrial fibrillation. The ventricular rate in this ECG is 30 bpm. The rhythm is irregularly irregular. No P waves are identified, but fibrillation (f) waves can be seen. The QRS-T complexes appear normal.

In Fig. 8.9B, the ventricular rate in this horse has increased to 50 bpm. No P waves can be identified, but there are more coarse fibrillation (or flutter) waves present (orange dashed arrows). The QRS morphology is similar to that seen in Fig. 8.9A, but the QRS complexes are approximately 36% wider now, while the T waves are larger and wider.

This horse has been receiving quinidine sulfate (QS) therapy, in an attempt to convert the atrial fibrillation to normal sinus rhythm. This is the second day of therapy. Initially, QS was given every 2 h for five doses, with a sixth dose 8 h later. The horse did not convert on the first day, so on the second day, QS was given every 4 h for two additional doses. This ECG (Fig. 8.9B) was recorded before the eighth dose of QS was given.

During the second day of treatment, the horse received IV fluid therapy with potassium and magnesium supplementation. A single dose of IV digoxin was given in the morning before the QS. It is important to supplement fluid and electrolytes in horses undergoing prolonged QS therapy, as they are often inappetant and can become dehydrated.

When giving QS, it is important that no more than six doses be delivered at 2 h intervals. Most horses will convert after three to four doses. If the horse does not convert during this time, therapy can be continued at longer dosing intervals, provided there are no clinical signs of adverse effects or toxicity observed, until a total dose of 180 mg/kg is administered. If adverse effects or signs of toxicity are observed, then QS should be discontinued and immediate measures provided to avoid life-threatening consequences.

Figure 8.9C was recorded 1.5 h after the eighth dose of QS. Here, the ventricular rate is 80 bpm. No clear P waves are seen; the horse has not yet converted to sinus rhythm. The QRS complexes are 75% wider than before treatment, and the T waves are large and wide. A single R-on-T phenomenon is seen (green arrow).

This horse should be treated immediately with a combination of medications:

- Magnesium sulfate (2–6 mg/kg/min to a total dose of 55 mg/kg, or 27.5 g for a 500 kg horse). This is the treatment of choice for quinidine-induced torsade de pointes (wide QRS tachycardia).
- Sodium bicarbonate (1 mEq/kg IV, or 500 ml of an 8.4% sodium bicarbonate solution for a 500 kg horse). This will antagonize the sodium-channel blocking effects of QS.
- Lidocaine hydrochloride (0.25-0.5 mg/kg very slowly IV, up to 1.5 mg/kg total dose over 10–15 min, or up to 750 mg for a 500 kg horse)
- Check electrolytes and replace as necessary.

Despite initiation of this therapy, the ECG rapidly deteriorated, as seen in Fig. 8.9D. The green arrow represents the first R-on-T phenomenon seen in Fig. 8.9C. Initially, single R-on-T phenomena are seen (red dashed arrows) but the rhythm quickly becomes more unstable, and wide QRS tachycardia develops and the horse collapses (torsade de pointes; purple dashed line). Despite a brief period where the rhythm stabilizes with therapy, further R-on-T phenomena occur (pink dashed arrow) and the rhythm rapidly deteriorates into ventricular flutter, fibrillation and then cardiac arrest within 5 min of the first R-on-T phenomenon. Attempts to resuscitate the horse were unsuccessful.

With the benefit of hindsight, given the QRS widening seen on Fig. 8.9B, no further QS should have been administered. The horse did not show any other adverse effects up until this point. Therapeutic drug monitoring performed immediately after death revealed a QS concentration of 4.38 µg/ml, within the therapeutic range of 2–5 µg/ml. This case highlights the fact that it only takes a single short-coupled premature complex to destabilize the ventricular electrical activity and result in sudden death.

Case 10 Answer

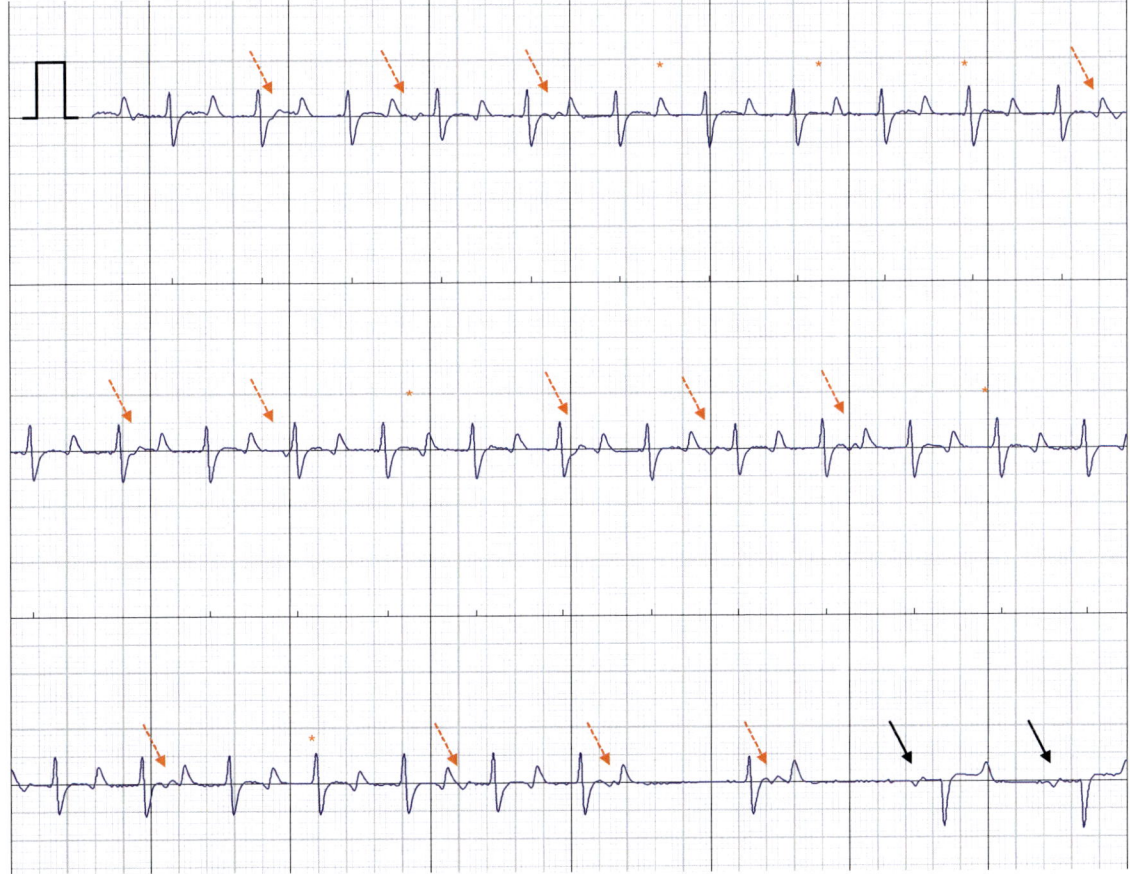

Fig. 8.10. ECG obtained using the AliveCor Kardia smartphone app. Paper speed: 25 mm/s.

This is an accelerated idioventricular rhythm or slow ventricular tachycardia. There are two sinus-origin complexes in the lower right-hand corner of the trace (black arrows). The remaining QRS complexes have a different morphology (RS) and are wider than the normal QRS complexes. P waves can be seen wandering in and out of the abnormal complexes (orange dashed arrows) indicating AV dissociation, but some P waves are more difficult to discern (orange asterisks). The ventricular rate is 100 bpm, while the atrial rate is 60 bpm.

Given the reduced clinical condition of the horse, this rhythm warrants immediate investigation. The following diagnostic evaluation was performed:

- Continuous telemetric ECG monitoring;
- Blood work to check electrolytes and cardiac troponin; and
- Echocardiography.

In addition, the horse was placed on IV fluid therapy, supplemented with magnesium sulfate (2–6 mg/kg/min to a total dose of 55 mg/kg, or 27.5 g for a 500 kg horse).

Echocardiography revealed a thickened ventricular myocardium, with dramatically reduced systolic and diastolic function. The pericardium was thickened, and consolidated lung could be seen immediately adjacent to the pericardium in the left thorax. No free pericardial fluid was seen. It was suspected that the pericardium and myocardium were inflamed secondary to the severe aspiration pneumonia. The cardiac troponin I was elevated (5 ng/ml).

Given the haemodynamic relevance of this ventricular rhythm, despite the relatively low rate, therapy with lidocaine hydrochloride (0.25–0.5 mg/kg very slowly IV, up to 1.5 mg/kg total dose over 10–15 min, or up to 750 mg for a 500 kg horse, followed by a continuous rate infusion of 0.05 mg/kg/min if necessary) is recommended to convert the rhythm back to sinus.

With this therapy, the ventricular rhythm slowed and then resolved over the next 4 h. The horse's clinical condition improved as the rhythm resolved. Additional non-steroidal anti-inflammatory medication was also given to reduce the inflammation associated with the aspiration pneumonia, pericarditis and myocarditis.

Echocardiography performed 1 week later showed improved myocardial function and reduced pericardial thickening, although the lung lesions took several months of therapy to fully resolve.

Accelerated idioventricular rhythms are commonly identified in horses with underlying systemic disease (e.g. systemic inflammatory response syndrome or haemorrhage). When the horse shows clinical signs of reduced perfusion (e.g. dull mentation, decreased appetite, poor jugular filling) or if multiple QRS morphologies or R-on-T phenomena are seen, then therapy with anti-arrhythmic medication is indicated. In addition, it is important to treat the underlying systemic disease.

References

Bers, D.M. (2002) Cardiac excitation-contraction coupling. *Nature* 415, 198–205.

Broux, B., de Clercq, D., Decloedt, A., van der Vekens, N., Verheyen, T. *et al.* (2016) Atrial premature depolarization-induced changes in QRS and T wave morphology on resting electrocardiograms in horses. *Journal of Veterinary Internal Medicine* 30, 1253–1259.

Broux, B., de Clercq, D., Decloedt, A., Ven, S., Vera, L. *et al.* (2017) Heart rate variability parameters in horses distinguish atrial fibrillation from sinus rhythm before and after successful electrical cardioversion. *Equine Veterinary Journal* 49, 723–728.

Buhl, R., Carstensen, H., Hesselkilde, E.Z., Klein, B.Z., Hougaard, K.M. *et al.* (2018) Effect of induced chronic atrial fibrillation on exercise performance in Standardbred trotters. *Journal of Veterinary Internal Medicine* 32, 1410–1419.

Decloedt, A., Schwarzwald, C.C., de Clercq, D., van der Vekens, N., Pardon, B. *et al.* (2015) Risk factors for recurrence of atrial fibrillation in horses after cardioversion to sinus rhythm. *Journal of Veterinary Internal Medicine* 29, 946–953.

Dong, J.G. (2016) The role of heart rate variability in sports physiology. *Experimental and Therapeutic Medicine* 11, 1531–1536.

Eggensperger, B.H. and Schwarzwald, C.C. (2017) Influence of 2nd-degree AV blocks, ECG recording length, and recording time on heart rate variability analyses in horses. *Journal of Veterinary Cardiology* 19, 160–174.

Flethoj, M., Kanters, J.K., Pedersen, P.J., Haugaard, M.M., Carstensen, H. *et al.* (2016) Appropriate threshold levels of cardiac beat-to-beat variation in semi-automatic analysis of equine ECG recordings. *BMC Veterinary Research* 12, 266.

Frick, L., Schwarzwald, C.C. and Mitchell, K.J. (2019) The use of heart rate variability analysis to detect arrhythmias in horses undergoing a standard treadmill exercise test. *Journal of Veterinary Internal Medicine* 33, 212–224.

Hamlin, R.L. and Smith, C.R. (1965) Categorization of common domestic mammals based upon their ventricular activation process. *Annals of the New York Academy of Sciences* 127, 195–203.

Heliczer, N., Gerber, V., Bruckmaier, R., van der Kolk, J.H. and de Solis, C.N. (2017) Cardiovascular findings in ponies with equine metabolic syndrome. *Journal of the American Veterinary Medical Association* 250, 1027–1035.

Jesty, S.A., Kraus, M.S., Johnson, A.L., Gelzer, A.R. and Bartol, J. (2011) An accessory bypass tract masked by the presence of atrial fibrillation in a horse. *Journal of Veterinary Cardiology* 13, 79–83.

Kinnunen, S., Laukkanen, R., Haldi, J., Hanninen, O. and Atalay, M. (2006) Heart rate variability in trotters during different training periods. *Equine Veterinary Journal* 38, 214–217.

Lenoir, A., Trachsel, D.S., Younes, M., Barrey, E. and Robert, C. (2017) Agreement between electrocardiogram and heart rate meter is low for the measurement of heart rate variability during exercise in young endurance horses. *Frontiers in Veterinary Science* 4, 170.

Luethy, D., Slack, J., Kraus, M.S., Gelzer, A.R., Habecker, P. and Johnson, A.L. (2017) Third-degree atrioventricular block and collapse associated with eosinophilic myocarditis in a horse. *Journal of Veterinary Internal Medicine* 31, 884–889.

Malik, M. *et al.* Task Force of the European Society of Cardiology/North Americam Society of Pacing Electrophysiology (1996) Heart rate variability: standards of measurement, physiological interpretation, and clinical use. *Circulation* 93, 1043–1065.

McConachie, E.L., Giguere, S., Rapoport, G. and Barton, M.H. (2016) Heart rate variability in horses with acute gastrointestinal disease requiring exploratory laparotomy. *Journal of Veterinary Emergency and Critical Care* 26, 269–80.

McGurrin, M.K., Physick-Sheard, P.W. and Kenney, D.G. (2008) Transvenous electrical cardioversion of equine atrial fibrillation: patient factors and clinical results in 72 treatment episodes. *Journal of Veterinary Internal Medicine* 22, 609–15.

Mitchell, K.J. (2019) Equine electrocardiography. *Veterinary Clinics: Equine Practice* 35, 65–83.

Ohmura, H., Hiraga, A., Aida, H., Kuwahara, M., Tsubone, H. and Jones, J.H. (2006) Changes in heart rate and heart rate variability in Thoroughbreds during prolonged road transportation. *American Journal of Veterinary Research* 67, 455–462.

Opie, L. (1998) *Heart Physiology from Cell to Circulation.* Lippincott-Raven, Philadelphia, Pennsylvania.

Pibarot, P., Vrins, A., Salmon, Y. and Difruscia, R. (1993) Implantation of a programmable atrioventricular pacemaker in a donkey with complete atrioventricular block and syncope. *Equine Veterinary Journal* 25, 248–251.

Reef, V.B. (2019) Assessment of the cardiovascular system in horses during prepurchase and insurance examinations. *Veterinary Clinics: Equine Practice* 35, 191–204.

Reef, V.B., Clark, E.S., Oliver, J.A. and Donawick, W.J. (1986) Implantation of a permanent transvenous pacing catheter in a horse with complete heart block and syncope. *Journal of the American Veterinary Medical Association* 189, 449–452.

Reef, V.B., Reimer, J.M. and Spencer, P.A. (1995) Treatment of atrial fibrillation in horses: new perspectives. *Journal of Veterinary Internal Medicine* 9, 57–67.

Reef, V.B., Bonagura, J., Buhl, R., McGurrin, M.K., Schwarzwald, C.C. *et al.* (2014) Recommendations for management of equine athletes with cardiovascular abnormalities. *Journal of Veterinary Internal Medicine* 28, 749–761.

Rietmann, T.R., Stauffacher, M., Bernasconi, P., Auer, J.A. and Weishaupt, M.A. (2004) The association between heart rate, heart rate variability, endocrine and behavioural pain measures in horses suffering from laminitis. *Journal of Veterinary Medicine A: Physiology, Pathology, Clinical Medicine* 51, 218–225.

Schwarzwald, C.C., Kedo, M., Birkmann, K. and Hamlin, R.L. (2012) Relationship of heart rate and electrocardiographic time intervals to body mass in horses and ponies. *Journal of Veterinary Cardiology* 14, 343–350.

Thayer, J.F., Hahn, A.W., Pearson, M.A., Sollers, J.J. 3rd, Johnson, P.J. and Loch, W.E. (1997) Heart rate variability during exercise in the horse. *Biomedical Sciences Instrumentation* 34, 246–251.

van Loon, G., Fonteyne, W., Rottiers, H., Tavernier, R. and Deprez, P. (2002) Implantation of a dual-chamber, rate-adaptive pacemaker in a horse with suspected sick sinus syndrome. *Veterinary Record* 151, 541–545.

van Steenkiste, G., de Clerq, D., Decloedt, A., Vera, L. and van Loon, G. (2018) Specific 12-lead ECG characteristics that help localize the anatomical origin of ventricular ectopy in horses: preliminary data. In: *Proceedings of the 11th European College of Equine Internal Medicine Congress*, 9–10 November 2018, Ghent, Belgium (abstract).

van Steenkiste, G., de Clercq, D., Vera, L., Decloedt, A. and van Loon, G. (2019) Sustained atrial tachycardia in horses and treatment by transvenous electrical cardioversion. *Equine Veterinary Journal* 51, 634–640.

Verheyen, T., Decloedt, A., van der Vekens, N., Sys, S., de Clercq, D. and van Loon, G. (2013) Ventricular response during lungeing exercise in horses with lone atrial fibrillation. *Equine Veterinary Journal* 45, 309–314.

Viu, J., Armengou, L., Decloedt, A. and Jose-Cunilleras, E. (2018) Investigation of ventricular pre-excitation electrocardiographic pattern in two horses: clinical presentation and potential causes. *Journal of Veterinary Cardiology* 20, 213–221.

von Borell, E., Langbein, J., Despres, G., Hansen, S., Leterrier, C. *et al.* (2007) Heart rate variability as a measure of autonomic regulation of cardiac activity for assessing stress and welfare in farm animals – a review. *Physiology & Behavior* 92, 293–316.

Woo, M.A., Stevenson, W.G., Moser, D.K., Trelease, R.B. and Harper, R.M. (1992) Patterns of beat-to-beat heart rate variability in advanced heart failure. *American Heart Journal* 123, 704–710.

Zuber, N., Zuber, M. and Schwarzwald, C.C. (2019) Assessment of systolic and diastolic function in clinically healthy horses using ambulatory acoustic cardiography. *Equine Veterinary Journal* 51, 391–400.

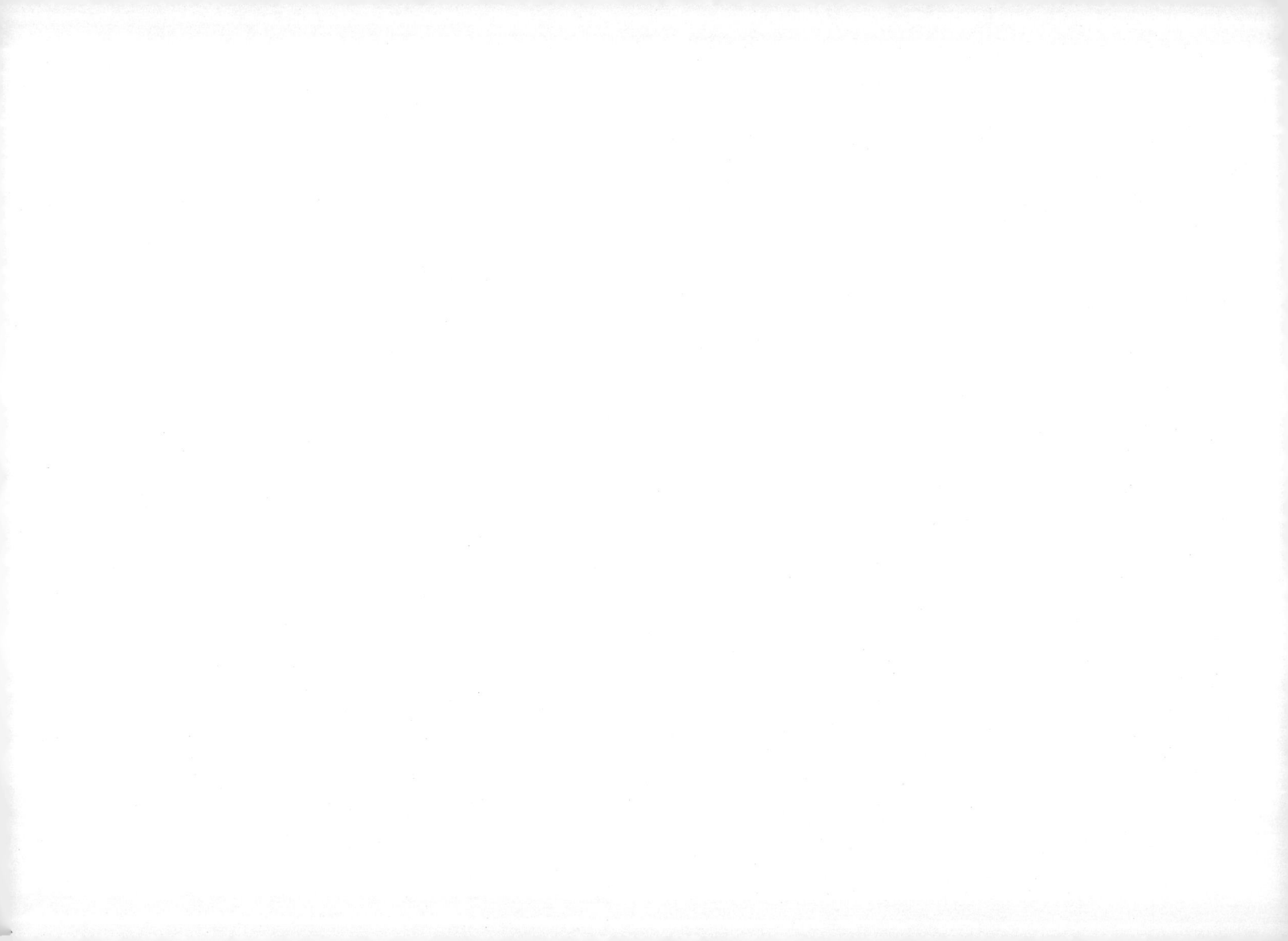

Index

Page numbers in **bold** type refer to figures, tables and boxed text.